So, Why Become Vegan?

☐ A. Nutritional Reasons
☐ B. Spiritual Reasons
☐ C. Environmental Reasons
☐ D. Ethical Reasons
☑ E. All of the Above

Sandra Kimler

BALBOA.
PRESS
A DIVISION OF HAY HOUSE

Balboa Press books may be ordered through booksellers or by contacting:

Balboa Press
A Division of Hay House
1663 Liberty Drive
Bloomington, IN 47403
www.balboapress.com.au
1 (877) 407-4847

Because of the dynamic nature of the Internet, any web addresses or
links contained in this book may have changed since publication and may
no longer be valid. The views expressed in this work are solely those
of the author and do not necessarily reflect the views of the publisher,
and the publisher hereby disclaims any responsibility for them.

The author of this book does not dispense medical advice or prescribe the
use of any technique as a form of treatment for physical, emotional, or medical
problems without the advice of a physician, either directly or indirectly. The
intent of the author is only to offer information of a general nature to help you
in your quest for emotional and spiritual well-being. In the event you use any
of the information in this book for yourself, which is your constitutional right,
the author and the publisher assume no responsibility for your actions.

Any people depicted in stock imagery provided by Thinkstock are models,
and such images are being used for illustrative purposes only.
Certain stock imagery © Thinkstock.

Printed in the United States of America.

ISBN: 978-1-4525-1373-7 (sc)
ISBN: 978-1-4525-1374-4 (e)

Balboa Press rev. date: 04/15/2014

I humbly dedicate this book
to all animal beings.
May you go in love, dignity and peace.

Contents

Preface ix

Gratitude xiii

PART ONE

Becoming More Aware 3

Inner Happiness and Ego 17

Consciousness 25

PART TWO

Nutrition and Veganism 39

    Soil 40

    The Alkaline and Acidic Diet 42

    Chemical Elements 47

    Iridology 66

    My own story 86

    Comparisons 90

    What Is Making You Unwell? 97

    Stress and Proper Digestion 101

    How to have a healthy bowel 104

    Better Out than In 107

    Emotional Ties with Your Food 108

Foodless Food..114

Abattoirs..121

Raw Food...124

Dairy Products..127

Allergies...135

Sandra's Super Foods..140

Kids' Lunchbox Fillers...147

Rainbow Salad...150

Spirituality and Veganism...155

Spiritual Growth...155

Meditation..157

Why Vegetarians Go Back to Eating Meat..................161

Ego..164

Breaking the Habit...167

Food Vibrations...173

Environment and Veganism...179

Unsustainability...179

Ethics and Veganism...189

Ethics and the Abattoir...189

Last word...195

PART THREE

Little Truths..207

Sandra's Super Banana Milkshake Recipe.......................243

Recommended Books..245

Recommended Documentaries...247

Recommended Websites..249

Famous Vegans..251

References...253

About the Author..255

Preface

So, why did I become a vegan? I must have been asked this question a thousand times over the years. The truth is, I feel that I've always been a vegan. I grew up in a normal, middle-class, nuclear family that ate meat and three veg at dinner. I can't say that I disliked meat. Both my parents were great cooks, and it was always a positive and cosy experience sitting around the table at 5 p.m. for dinner.

I grew up in Rotterdam in the Netherlands, and my interactions with animals were very limited. It was not until I was taken to a Kids Animal Farm around the age of five that the penny dropped. That night, my family had a very different experience around the dinner table, as I questioned my parents' feeding choices. My parents' relaxed attitude to the idea of an animal having to be killed so we could eat it left me dumbfounded. I remember feeling scared of my parents for a moment, almost expecting a monster to jump out of their bodies and say "Gotcha! Yes, we've made you eat animals and you didn't even know it!" I honestly thought something was seriously wrong with them. I could not believe they had fed me this stuff without consulting me first. This feeling stayed with me for a while. I felt betrayed because I had not been given a choice.

My parents light-heartedly explained that this was what humans did, that we must eat meat in order to be healthy, that it was an acceptable practice, and everyone did it.

Their argument did not convince me. I just felt it was the wrong thing to do, yet I was required to eat meat. At that age, I did not know how to disobey my parents or stand up for myself. I told them I did not want to eat meat anymore, and that was when "dinner" became a not-so-cosy experience. My hatred of eating meat grew to such an extent that I ended up winning the war. One night when I was around ten years old, we had meatballs for dinner, and once again I asked my parents if I could leave the meat; once again the answer was no! I don't know what came over me, but I picked up a meatball, sauce and all, and threw it across the room, leaving a trail of red sauce on my parents' furniture and the carpet before it came to a halt. I knew I was the next "dead meat" now and that my father wanted to throw me across the room, so I stood up to receive my deserved punishment. My father stood up with a red face ready to explode. And then it happened: —my mother gently touched my father's arm and said, "Sit down. From now on, she will not have to eat meat again."

I quietly cleaned up the mess, avoiding eye contact with my father, but inside I was cheering in triumph, laughing and jumping for joy. I realised the phenomenon that had just occurred.

Over time, my brother, my mother, and yes, almost my father became vegetarians.

Thirty-five years later, while walking on a beach in Bali, a friend asked me, "So, why did you become a vegan?" It was at that moment I thought to write this book. The answer to that question is a combination of everything I had come to understand in my life. These understandings are mine and mine alone. They are based on the research I have done over the last twenty-five years. I worked in the health and healing industry with my mum, who started this study of nutrition, spiritual awakening, meditation, awareness, humbleness, gratefulness and forgiveness before me.

All my mum's findings led many women who came to her "Skin and Beauty Care Centre" to a happy, balanced, and healthy life. It didn't matter who came for treatment; the healing process became predictable for every client.

I was fortunate to work and study closely with my mum. She was my mentor, teacher and employer, but most of all she was my dearest mum, my friend who knew me so well and loved me unconditionally. I often wondered how much knowledge has been lost because she passed over. She was able to tell you what you ate and drank the night before, just by looking at the colour of your skin. She could tell you what kind of diet you had for the year, just by looking at the colour of your eyes, and she could tell you what kind of person you were and what kind of life you had led by touching your hands and feeling the stiffness or suppleness of your fingers. One thing was always certain: she could heal you using correct eating habits, meditation and forgiveness.

My mother's research showed clearly that in order to be healthy and vibrant, we needed an alkaline body and peace of mind. One could not get better without the health of the other. One would toxify the other if one wasn't corrected. People responded identically to this balanced way of life and became better in body, mind and spirit.

This book will share some of the teachings and little wisdoms that I have inherited from my mum. It is full of borrowed material. I can tell you that 80 percent of what I have written came from the mouths of or was guided by the actions of two teachers: my mum, Hennie Spykers-Hersman, and Dr. Bernard Jensen. I've attended many of Dr. Jensen's lectures, which reflect the teachings that appear in his books. Another 10 percent is from my own "aha" moments, and 10 percent is from everyone else's findings.

The health and well-being of all living creatures is based on the choices we make. A vegan lifestyle is as cruelty-free as possible, environmentally friendly and extremely healthy. If you have ever wanted to flirt with veganism or questioned the path you are on, this book will take you on a confronting and informative journey from which you may not want to return.

I hope you enjoy it. Take the bits and pieces you can use for your own growth. Take notes, read sections again and put it into practice. Feel free to use any material in this book for your own use. I sincerely hope that the contents of this book will stimulate your thoughts and challenge old belief patterns and habits.

Allow your awareness to expand, and the path will appear and so might the question—So, why become vegan?

> *"The sick have just one wish and the healthy have many."*
> —*Indian Proverb*

Gratitude

I want to express my gratitude to Oprah for the many "aha" moments. To Ellen for your generosity. To Lyn White for being the voice for animals. To Dr. Bernard Jensen for providing the stepping stones to guide my life's journey. To Wilson Luna, who always said "Live, Love, Contribute." To my mother, Hennie, for being my twin soul. No words can describe what you have given to me and others. It was a privilege to be your daughter. I also express gratitude to my children, Lee, Kye, and Kelsey, for whom I joyously rise each day.

I want to thank my loving husband, Dierk Kimler, for his patience while helping me put this book together. I could not have done this without you.

Part One

Becoming More Aware

A vegetarian eats no food that directly required an animal to be killed to consume them. A vegetarian may still eat dairy, eggs, honey, rennet and gelatine. If you eat fish, you are *not* a vegetarian; you are a pescatarian. You eat no meat and poultry, but you do eat fish and seafood. Vegetarianism is the practice of excluding all animal flesh, including fish, seafood, crustaceans, game and poultry. Veganism is far stricter. It is a lifestyle, rather than a dietary choice. A vegan's primary focus is to be compassionate to all animals.

A dietary vegan does not eat anything that has an animal product in it. An ethical vegan follows a vegan diet and also includes the vegan philosophy in every aspect of his or her life. Vegans do not wear fur, leather, wool or silk. They do not use products that have been tested on animals. They do not condone hunting, fishing, dog or horseracing, medical testing, on animals, circus animals and zoos.

> "One should not wish to benefit from that which does not belong to him."
>
> —Author unknown.

When people ask me, "What made you a vegan?" I say that I feel that I was born that way. What made you a meat eater? Think about it. We are born vegans, and it is our parents who conditioned us to eat meat. We are taught from a very early age *what* to think, rather than *how to think for ourselves.* Take a moment to visualise yourself walking through the woods. You are enjoying the peacefulness and feeling close to nature. You see a squirrel. What is your reaction? "Oh, how cute is that!" is a normal response. As you walk on, you see a blackberry bush. What is your reaction? "Yum." Our instinct is to pick the berries and eat them. Our natural instinct never made us want to eat the squirrel. Think about it.

Have you ever observed a child's behaviour at a kids' animal farm? Parents take their children to such places so that they can pat and feed the calves, lambs and chickens. The children, in their own special way, want to be kind to the animals. They have this need to hold them. It is almost an obsessive behaviour. Hopefully, for the animals' sake, the parents will guide the child how to be gentle in their loving handling of the animal. Their need to be connected with the animal being is very strong. It is like they need to be with an animal's life force. Why is it that children so badly want a dog, or a cat, a guinea pig or some kind of animal to love? It is their natural instinct to want to be connected with an animal's life force.

If we would ask a child holding a chick at the animal farm, "Would you like to eat this chick?", what do you think the child would say? The child probably wouldn't say much, because he would be in shock. Tears would well up in his eyes and he would run to his parents, crying, "Mum, this woman wants me to eat a chicken!" Well, my guess is that the child already does eat chicken, and it was his parents who cleverly disguised it as mince or satay, or a slice on his bread. In childhood, once our bodies and taste buds are accustomed to eating meat, we grow up as meat-eaters, wondering how those crazy "vegos" do it. After all, we are meant to eat meat, aren't we?

> *"Teaching a child not to step on a caterpillar is as valuable to the child as it is to the caterpillar."*
>
> *—Bradley Miller*

Do you have any memories from when you were a child, of walking through the vegetable patch with an adult, picking beans, strawberries and tomatoes? If the answer is yes, how did it feel? If the answer is no, how do you think it would have felt? Good, right?

Now, do you have any childhood memories of an adult taking you through an abattoir—a slaughterhouse? If the answer is no, how do you think it would feel? If the answer is yes, you are probably a vegan fighting for animal rights. So what changes? As children, our bodies are pure, with pure, clean cells.

It is our parents who introduce death to us in the form of cooked meat. It is heavily disguised with salt, spices and sauces, in shapes, as deep-fried food or on a barbeque, dripping in tomato sauce. In nature, all omnivores and carnivores eat their meat raw. Eating raw and bloody meat is disgusting to us, so we cook and season it. Human meat-eaters do anything to get rid of the raw-meat taste. How do you think raw meat would taste? Our palate would not approve. As we grow, our cells slowly lose their pureness, and our taste buds take over, as we become detached from the animals we were once so fondly connected to. Eating meat is considered an ethical, moral and traditional issue. To go against any of this is like an insult to our mothers. We even make up excuses for the slaughter of animal beings. We say things like: "We need animal protein", and "we need iron." "God created animals for our use" and even, "We must take the life force of a goat by slicing open her neck while facing Mecca; otherwise we don't go to heaven".

Who made up those rules? What about: Thou shalt not kill? or "Do to others what you would like for yourself". It clearly doesn't apply to animal beings.

How about: Wish for others what you would wish for yourself? For example: shelter, food, kindness, no fear and a safe place to reproduce naturally. Sorry, we say, this only applies to human beings, not animal beings. The men who made up these rules all those centuries ago must have really known their stuff. They clearly separated the needs of humans from the needs of animal beings.

What about our dogs and cats? Would you eat them? Why not? Is it because you have an emotional and physical attachment to them? Well, people do eat dogs in places where they don't eat cows because of their attachment to the cow.

Can you see that we make up all these rules to suit ourselves? This is why there are whale lovers and whale-meat lovers. Why is the killing of a whale more horrific than the killing of a cow? Well, because we want to watch them in our oceans. We are attached to what our needs are. Lucky whale! In some parts of the world, horsemeat is eaten. Instead of Pony Club, they have pony club sandwiches.

There are patterns in human behaviour, and they are all taught when we are young children. We learn to attach ourselves to what we are told our needs are, and we learn to detach for the same reason.

> *"People often say that humans have always eaten animals, as if this is a justification for continuing the practice. According to this logic, we should not try to prevent people from murdering other people, since this has also been done since the earliest of times."*
>
> *—Isaac Bashevis Singer (1902–1991)*

We consider the image of Jesus suffering on the cross to be significant because we can relate to it. We wouldn't want to be in his sandals. We can identify with his suffering. What about the suffering of animal beings? How do we relate to that? Maybe we should start by being aware of the suffering caused by human hands. For instance, we can relate to the fact that animals need shelter, just like we do. They also need food naturally suited for their bodies. Mad cow disease occurred because the cows' feed consisted of pellets made from animal protein. This was an unnecessary cruelty brought on by ignorant humans. Animal beings are very good mothers. Have you ever seen the panic in a cow's eyes when her calf is taken away? I know that human mothers could relate to this if they imagined their child being taken away. For weeks, a cow will call out for her calf while being milked by something that does not resemble her child.

Maybe all of this is on a different level, but animal beings would be so much happier if they were allowed to live a life without human interference.

People will argue that we need cow's milk for the calcium. The cow would argue that she eats greens to get her calcium! Besides that, humans are the only mammal that drinks milk past the age of two. Humans are also the only mammal that drinks milk from an other species. In simple terms, our systems are designed to absorb calcium from human milk only when we're small infants. After that, we become lactose intolerant. Yes, all of us over the age of two are lactose intolerant. Our bodies cannot absorb milk, and it is no longer a food. Instead, milk and dairy products will cause a huge amount of mucus, which the body can't expel quickly enough, resulting in asthma, sinus problems, coughing, bronchitis, tonsillitis, earaches, snotty noses, sluggishness and in general an acidic, unhealthy body.

> *"I've never had a sinus infection or been on antibiotics since cutting out dairy."*
>
> *—Mayim Bialik, actress and neuroscientist*

Once we make the connection that the suffering of an animal being is directly linked to our behavioural needs, it becomes easier to change ourselves. Once we give up "suffering-causing actions," instinctively you'll know you have done the right thing. A beautiful energy appears inside us. It might be small at first, but it is a new beginning nevertheless. We might even become aware of how much animal beings have suffered at our hands, directly and indirectly. Slowly but surely, our inner self will change. We become more aware, passionate and understanding. This ability to relate better will overflow to all parts of our life. Ultimately, this will influence those around us, spreading out to all parts of the world. Now *that* is where the connection is. We are connecting on a global-awareness level. Once our mental state has changed, our physical bodies will change as well.

Our cells will begin to change. They will become pure, just like when we were young, but even more so, because now we are conscious of this change. We in turn will feel enlightened when we understand that our actions towards our fellow beings— human as well as animal—have a direct effect on us. We can no longer do harm because we will know that doing so will harm ourselves. Our lives will change because of the difference in our behaviour. We will perceive and observe things differently. We go to a friend's barbeque like we've done so many times before, and we notice the men standing around, doing their thing. We look at the steak being thrown on the barbeque, covered in salt and pepper. People are laughing, drinking, poking the meat with their barbeque fork, and having a good time.

The difference is that this time, we'll notice that the very being we once were so connected to is disrespectfully burning on a rack of filth. This is what people eat. Have you ever smelled lamb odour coming from a human? I guarantee that they ate it the night before. Every cell of their body will want to expel this meat quickly. The odour coming from a vegan is clean. No need for deodorizers, perfumes or Odor Eaters in shoes. Did you know that when a vegan reaches orgasm, it smells sweet? It is clean because a vegan eats clean.

> "I have from an early age abjured the use of meat, and the time will come when men such as I look upon the murder of animals as they now look upon the murder of men."
> —Leonardo da Vinci

What you give out, you get back three times over, and your lovemaking is an extension of the life that is within you. It is as wholesome, as the life you lead. So how do we change? How do we begin this cell-cleansing process?

We make the decision in our head first, and the rest will follow. Start by saying no to unwholesome foods. Don't buy them. Don't bring it into your home. Go easy on yourself. Realize that we are forever changing and evolving. The biggest obstacle here is knowing the right thing to do and then not doing it. It doesn't take long for our bodies to adjust and not want to go back to old habits. You are always learning. Let the new become the old, and let it go. Then embrace the next level. Replace meat with organic tofu, but not tofu products that taste like meat. Include lentils, brown rice, legumes, nuts and seeds in your diet. All of these are very high in protein that the body can easily absorb. Start reading books on the subject. Kathy Freston's book *Veganist* and *Fit for Life* by Marilyn Diamond are both wonderful.

> *"And check this out: If every American had one meat-free day per week, it would be the same as taking eight million cars off American roads in a year."*
>
> —*Kathy Freston*

Vegan cookbooks are the best because they don't include any animal products. Eat at vegan/vegetarian restaurants; Hare Krishna restaurants are great and very affordable. Become aware of all the live food that is available to you. Maybe you could grow some veggies yourself. Go to vegan and vegetarian websites to educate yourself. Pick out the information you can use. Don't go overboard. Enjoy the change, but also observe the change within yourself. Brush your skin with a loofah made of natural fibres. Wake up those cells! Those who eat death have dead cells. Drink plenty of water. Lead by example. Don't preach to people rather show them by setting an example. The key to an easy relationship with other people is not to impose your opinion or crush the opinion of others. Everyone is on his or her own path, with his or her own belief systems. I once knew of a priest who said, "I cringe at the thought of what I used to preach. Even I don't believe that stuff anymore." The Dalai Lama said, "There are over 6.5 billion people in the world and there should be as many different belief systems."

Not only are we all different from each other, but because we change constantly, we live our lives according to what we believe at that moment.

Bring your focus to yourself and your changes, not others. Only talk about your changes when asked. When the student is ready, a teacher will appear. Be that teacher. It is, of course, advisable to tell those close around you what you are about to do. Allow them to have their own opinion. This is your truth. Maybe they will support your journey and maybe they'll even feel like a change as well. You can hope for a positive reaction from your family and friends, but recognise that they have their own path. You have planted a seed. Stand back and watch it grow. People will notice the difference in you. They will say, "Gee, you look good," or "Have you been on a holiday?" The lines in your face will soften. Your muscles will tone. You will walk lighter. Your bowels will function better. You will lose weight. Meat is so hard to digest. It putrefies our system because our intestines are way too long to expel meat quickly. The intestines of natural meat-eaters like lions, cats and dogs are very short. They eat and expel the meat before it becomes putrid. Our bodies are thirty-seven degrees Celsius. That is pretty hot.

Next time it is this hot on a summer's day, put a steak outside in the sun. On average, meat takes twenty-four hours to digest at this temperature. Observe how quickly the meat goes off and starts smelling. The stench becomes so bad that you will have to remove it before the sun goes down. So, you can see that in our human digestive system, big lumps of meat just sit there, rotting away. If we finally eat a green salad to move it along, when the meat finally comes out the other end, it will stink, just like dog poo does, and we cannot use it for compost. However, human vegan poo does not smell so bad, and I put it in my garden along with chicken poo. Vegan poo starts out as green life energy, and from it you can grow other green life energies. Poo that started as a suffering animal being intoxicated by adrenaline and fear is so revolting that worms, the life force of this earth, will not go anywhere near it. Yet in vegan poo, they happily multiply.

"We are the living graves of murdered beasts, slaughtered to satisfy our appetites. How can we hope in this world to attain the peace we say we are so anxious for?"

—George Bernard Shaw
(Living Graves, published 1951)

So how does that relate to the energy of a person? Are they aware of the low vibrations they are putting out—or should I say "pushing out"? Do low-energy people lead an ignorant life? Do low-energy people watch violent movies without feeling bad because they are on the same energy level? They can watch horrific news stories on TV and not feel affected. Perhaps they can read about tragedies in the newspaper and think nothing of it and not be affected because they have the same energy level as these negative stories.

As our diet changes, we change, and with that our energy changes. We cannot watch horror or violent movies. It makes us feel sick because of the negative energy. Negative people start to affect us, and we voluntarily stay away from these people. We start watching gardening shows, or we stop watching TV altogether. We start reading books, and we stop negative activities such as duck hunting.

These might be small changes, but inside, our vibrations will also change. We'll start communicating with our children without aggression. We'll recognise when other parents are stressed, and we won't judge them.

> "Flesh-eating by humans is unnecessary, irrational, anatomically unsound, unhealthy, unhygienic, uneconomic, unaesthetic, unkind and unethical. May I elaborate?"
> —Helen Nearing, Simple Food for the Good Life

We begin to enjoy simple pleasures. We find out that when we change ourselves, the people around us also change. Eventually we become at ease with being on a higher level. All of a sudden, we don't want to go to Maccy D's. We'd rather have a salad sandwich and eat it in the park while watching children playing and squirrels relishing the leftover food. You notice a mother duck attending to her twelve ducklings ever so thoroughly, and you share your bread with her. It gives you a warm, fuzzy feeling.

Imagine, then, that you see an overtired mother punish her unruly child by smacking him. Instead of judging her, you'll understand her struggle but will also take special notice of a Maccy D's bag and a Coke next to the child. You'll realize your opinions have softened and that, perhaps, not so long ago you were like that parent. Now you take your child to a health café, where he eats a salad wrap and drinks a freshly squeezed juice. There is no playground at the health café, so you spend time talking with your child. You find out that he is having some problems at school. That night, instead of shooshing him during the evening news, you turn off the TV and talk about his problems at school.

> "You ask people why they have deer heads on the wall. They always say, 'Because it's such a beautiful animal.' There you go. I think my mother's attractive, but I have photographs of her."
>
> —Ellen DeGeneres

The changes are small and subtle. On the weekend, you go to a barbeque, and you notice that as your friends drink alcohol, their energy levels change. You decide to have a small glass of bubbly, just to be polite, but really you could have done without it. You all eat sausages, and you feel you could have done without them. You decide that next time you're going to say "no thanks"—if there is a next time.

You enrol in a basic massage course; you feel that the energy is different here. The conversation is different; it is on a different level. The women talk about how they could easily be vegans if it weren't for their husbands' meat-eating habits. One woman suggests replacing meat with tofu. A light goes on in your head. In fact, so many lights have been going on lately. I call them "aha" moments. A lot to think about.

The next time you have coffee with your girlfriends, you want to talk about your experiences, but all your girlfriends seem to be interested in is gossip. Has it always been that way? The next time you meet your friends, you feel out of place. You try to strike up a conversation about forest conservation, but it falls on deaf ears because the footy team had their second loss in a row and there is a lot to whinge about.

You feel youself growing apart from these people. You no longer laugh at their sexist jokes because you now hear how disrespectful these are towards your sisters. This reminds me of what a friend once said to me: "If you met your old friends today, would you want to befriend them?" What a good question. The change in our thinking clearly shows that we are on an evolving path. Some of us evolve faster than others, and therefore we grow apart from each other. Sometimes we can reconnect, and sometimes we lovingly let people go. The path to the top is often travelled alone but not lonely. You travel only with equals, and if there is no one, you travel alone.

So how does this relate to being a vegan? It all has to do with vibrations. We only attract people and situations on the same vibrational level, give or take a frequency of two. The less suffering you bring to others, the more compassionate you will feel. In order to feel peace, you must let go of anger. This leads to laughter and forgiveness. You learn to have trust in what you *feel,* not in what you *know.* Wisdom comes when we let go of what we know. Our stomach softens, and we digest better. We start drinking more water. Our depression is lessened; in fact, we feel a hint of inner peace. The next time you decide to eat meat, it sits like a rock in your stomach. This level of vibration does not agree with you any longer.

> "If any kid ever realized what was involved in factory farming, they would never touch meat again. I was so moved by the intelligence, sense of fun and personalities of the animals I worked with on Babe that by the end of the film, I was a vegetarian."
>
> —James Cromwell

Inner Happiness and Ego

Self-knowledge leads to a higher level of vibration, which leads to inner happiness, which leads to a change in cells, which leads to wanting to be healthier, which leads to a higher awareness of what to put in your mouth. This leads to an environment of well-being.

Ignorance becomes obsolete. One must know oneself. Everything becomes clearer. You are no longer what you always believed you were. Everything that was the norm we now question, like old habits, old belief systems, and the way we lived and ate. We cannot go backwards to the old. The new is light, and life actually feels easier. It seems like a natural evolution of life, as we happily implement these changes in our lives. We are not stuck.

We swap our romantic book club for yoga classes, and then we learn to meditate. This is when the wheel of life becomes the wheel of the divine. We start reading spiritual books, as we hunger for inner knowledge. We become more intuitive for example, when our child comes home, we instinctively feel we should comfort him because of his troublesome day.

You explain to your child that bullies are a product of their own environment, and together you send this bully some loving thoughts and wish a kind voice for him when he gets home from school.

> *"Throughout life people will make you mad, disrespect you and treat you bad. Let God deal with the things they do, cause hate in your heart will consume you too."*
>
> —*Will Smith*

The vibration has shifted. That night, your partner comments on what a lovely feel the house has. You have soft music on. There are some candles displayed, and the atmosphere is kind. You feed your family a vegan meal. It is easy digestible. For once, you don't want to flop on the couch in front of the TV because you're exhausted after eating a lump of negativity for dinner. Your family talks for a while, laughs, and enjoys each other's company after dinner.

We connect and reconnect with all that is good over and over again. Our conscious awareness is awakened. You become responsible for your actions. How can you inflict pain to anyone, human and animal, directly or indirectly? This is *conscious awakening!*

Do you think this transaction will go smoothly? No way! Unfortunately, this is where the ego kicks in. The ego has a very low energy. It is controlling and dominating and needs to be in power with all its might. The ego never wants to change; change is its enemy. The ego plays an important role in the human saga. People will openly show their anger. They'll fight tooth and nail to protect the belief systems instilled by their parents and reinforced by their ego. Partners will show anger towards changes because of the loss of control they feel. They feel threatened—or rather it is their ego that stops them from just going with the flow.

Generally, women find change easier to deal with as women's egos aren't as deeply embedded as men's. This is particularly true for women who have children, as they know what it means to devote themselves to others. Even when they're exhausted, they find the energy to get up at night to feed their children. Women also take care of the elderly in larger numbers than men. This also speaks to their abilities to put others' needs before their own. Of course, many men have these qualities as well. In fact, more and more men are changing. More and more husbands happily change nappies, share household duties, and have equal input into the upbringing of their children with their partners, seeing their relationships as partnerships rather than hierarchies.

> *"Fairness does not mean everyone gets the same. Fairness means everyone gets what they need."*
>
> *—Rick Riordan*

This change is happening all over the world. There is a global awareness happening. This is not a new thing; it has been happening since man first walked upright. The obvious changes are: we no longer burn women at the stake, the abolition of slavery in Western countries, children's rights, animal rights, women's rights, gay rights, acceptance of the evolution theory, pollution awareness, and acknowledgement of Native Indian and Aboriginal laws. We now say "sorry" for the injustice men have put on these people. It was their egos that made them feel superior. These men felt it was their right to act this way. Their laws only benefitted themselves. Imagine being the first person to try to change these men. Change is not easy, but as people become more enlightened, it becomes obvious that we've been on the wrong path for far too long. Not so obvious is that we need to let go of our ego. *Men* need to let go of their status. To truly change, people need to let go of status and communicate rather than forcing their views on others.

> *"Nothing will benefit human health and increase chances for survival of life on Earth as much as the evolution to a vegetarian diet."*
>
> —Albert Einstein, *quoted in* Sinfully Vegan

The men who have the greatest difficulty with change are those whose beliefs are deeply embedded. They wholeheartedly feel that a woman is beneath them. To them, it is nothing to beat, rape or kill a woman. Belief systems are often endorsed by religion. Even in Christianity, we find women struggling for equal rights. And who has a problem with equal rights? That's right: men. It's men's egos that see women's power as a threat to their own. Even outside knowledge is a threat. TV has shown men in vulnerable situations, showing compassion, fall in love and change nappies. For those men who are open to change, it will bring a change to what would otherwise be a rigid community. Slowly but surely, there is a change on a global scale and level. There is an energy shift. When people feel threatened, they become angry.

I feel that we have increased the planet's awareness vibration. The earth's aura has gone from black to grey, and many people are on the doorstep of a higher level of consciousness.

> "The possibility of stepping into a higher plane is quite real for everyone. It requires no force or effort or sacrifice. It involves little more than changing our ideas about what is normal."
> —Deepak Chopra

Global consciousness will keep on evolving in the right direction. People will become more aware of the suffering that goes on around them, but most importantly, they will want to stop the suffering they are causing themselves. How environmentally aware were we fifty years ago, even ten or five years ago? On the whole, we've become very aware of the suffering we've caused. How far will we go to reverse this suffering? Our governments would have to let go of their egos and share their wealth with all humans. We would stop deforestation, respect different religions and stop using animals for our own needs. In fact, the list is way too long, but we can start with ourselves. We could put carbon footprints on the top of the list of importance. How much pollution did I cause by using this product? How far did it have to travel? How many trees were needed to make it? You could holiday in your own area, drive hybrid cars, and stop buying products that cause the raping of this Earth. Buy local, organically grown food; the list goes on.

All of these things are already in place, but it will take a greater awareness to make them common. In another five years, this list will be much larger as global conscious awareness has grown.

> *"We need a new environmental consciousness on a global basis. To do this, we need to educate people."*
> —*Mikhail Gorbachev*

When a positive change has occurred, no matter how small, we feel the godliness within ourselves. As we see the goodness within ourselves, we recognise the good in others. It humbles us to see how much we still have to learn. We want to surround ourselves with those we can learn from, those who have wisdom and practice what they preach. We understand that we all are on the path of inner knowledge. We are not separated from each other, and we recognize those people whose ego stops them from this wonderful experience.

We respect people who give of themselves, those who live their lives respecting the Earth. Their joy is in knowing they don't bring ignorant suffering. These people make their homes more environmentally friendly, replant forests, join activist groups, donate to orphanages or animal shelters. It doesn't matter where their passion lies; it all helps to reduce suffering. How does that compare with those who do not connect on this level? The question is, why don't they? I feel it is because of their ego. They are still too self-centred to perform actions that don't specifically benefit them. They'll climb Mt Everest, but who did they serve when conquering the mountain?

> *"The measure of a man is how he behaves when no one is looking."*
>
> *—Wilson Luna.*

Why are acts like these glorified? They are glorified only by those who have the same vibration as those who are doing the act. Those with wealth are in a position to do great things for our planet. It can be hard to be humble, but this is their karma. How wonderful it is to see the results of their efforts when they put their money to good use and what a pity when they don't take this opportunity to donate to the world. These people donate to their own egos. And that is all I'm going to say about that!

> *"I believe that hope for the future depends on each of us taking nonviolence into our hearts and minds and developing new and imaginative structures which are nonviolent and life-giving for all. Some people will argue that this is too idealistic. I believe it is very realistic. I am convinced that humanity is fast evolving to this higher consciousness. For those who say it cannot be done, let us remember that humanity learned to abolish slavery. Our task now is no less than the abolition of violence and war... We can rejoice and celebrate today because we are living in a miraculous time. Everything is changing and everything is possible."*
>
> *—Mairead Corrigan Maguire*

Consciousness

Not long ago, I was at a building site, and I was astonished by the personal rubbish that was around from the various builders: food scraps, bar wrappers, plastic cans, sandwich bags, cigarette butts and empty packets. I expressed my concern, and I was told that this wasn't bad at all compared to other building sites. I told them they missed my point. I was amazed that there were still people out there who were comfortable enough to rubbish our Earth.

It was the mentality of these people, the lack of respect and the level of consciousness. Again I was told this wasn't bad, and really what was the big deal, as the building site will be cleaned up when finished in five months' time. Okay, maybe I'd better give them an example to simplify the point I was trying to make. Ten years ago, we as a nation were comfortable throwing things out of the car window while we were driving— an apple core here, a cigarette butt there, a wrapper or a chewy. (If you are one of these rare people who didn't do this, I apologize for this generalization.) We were fairly unconscious in that respect.

"And we're seeing a higher level of consciousness and many more opportunities for people to challenge their present ways of thinking and move into a grander and larger experience of who they really are."

—Neale Donald Walsch

Compare that to today. Most Australians will feel outraged when we catch someone rubbishing while driving. We feel obliged to report them, and they will get a fine. We talk bad about these people, saying, "What's wrong with them?" We might even stop the car and pick up their rubbish. We feel we did the right thing for the day. The people who rubbish so easily are not conscious of the fact that what they were doing was wrong. It is not their fault. Their ego makes it hard for them to change. These people simply don't think about their actions; if they did, that would be the first step towards change. Once people start thinking about their actions they most likely will try to justify what they do at first. but in time, they themselves find that they no longer justify those actions. They'll be conscious of what they do and will hold themselves accountable.

So, when I showed my disbelief at the building site, it was towards the lack of consciousness that was still within these people. I was not judging these individuals, for they didn't know what they did was wrong. I believe that people are generally good and don't want to hurt anyone or destroy things on purpose.

"No problem can be solved from the same level of consciousness that created it."

—Albert Einstein

As written in the bible, Jesus said, "Forgive them, Father, for they don't know what they have done." It was their lack of consciousness he was talking about. You cannot teach a two-year-old child algebra, and once you realize this, it is easier to understand and forgive people. At most, feel pity for the lack of awakening.

> Daniel and his friends refuse to eat from the king's table, which has meat on it, but eat vegetables instead. After ten days they are found to be healthier than those who eat at the king's table.
>
> (Daniel 1:3–16)

It is as much the ignorance of the unaware as it is the intolerance of the aware that creates disharmony in our world. There is a battle of egos between those who do the physical harming (as in polluting) and those who have intolerance (emotional harming) to these people. We must communicate on a level of harmony. Show change in actions. Change yourself, and those around you will change as well.

Everyone is on his or her own path, and small awakenings are happening all around the world, often simultaneously. Global consciousness is real, and it proves that we are all connected. Why is littering frowned upon in most countries in the world these days? Because a thought was put into action some time ago regarding recycling, reusing, forest protection, etc. We became aware that we had to stop destroying the Earth. The same feelings and ideas popped up all over the world around the same time.

"It is from numberless diverse acts of courage and belief that human history is shaped. Each time a man stands up for an ideal, or acts to improve the lot of others, or strikes out against injustice, he sends forth a tiny ripple of hope and daring. Those ripples build a current which can sweep down the mightiest walls of oppression and resistance."

—Robert F. Kennedy

So how does veganism fit into this? When I saw all that litter at the building site, it hurt me. It hurt me that someone could do this to our beautiful Earth, which is struggling so much already. I had to voice my opinion because the Earth cannot do it herself. For whose benefit was the site littered? The answer is the ego and laziness of man. I always ask that question when egos are involved and the victim cannot voice its case. "For whose benefit?" is a powerful question, and the answer is always crystal clear. All over the world, people ask this very same question, and they are on the side of the underdog, whether it is related to the environment, animal beings, poverty, or human abuse. The injustice and unfairness make our hair stand up. It hurts us inside to know its suffering. It's because of our global connection that suffering directly affects us. We can't feel good knowing something or someone we care about is suffering under human hands. Its low vibration makes us dizzy or even sick. It makes our blood boil to see a thousand-year-old tree being bulldozed and made into chips, exported for a miserable seven dollars per tonne. Yet it happens every day, but for how long? We feel sick and look away when a bull is stabbed to death in a bullfight, but it still happens every day, but for how long? We don't think dancing bears are cute, yet this cruelty happens every day, but for how long?

Those people who are waking up and becoming conscious, their behaviour becomes a conscious "doing." They cannot be a part of ignorant, destructive behaviour anymore.

So what about this next outrageous statement? "We are numb with disbelief to know animal beings are farmed in horrific conditions, only to be slaughtered in order to accompany our three veg." Yet it still happens… but for how much longer?

Just because you have believed something to be right for a long time, it doesn't mean you have to believe it forever. If you change your thinking, you'll change your life.

When someone becomes sick, they have a small window of opportunity to change for the better. They won't feel like smoking; they won't feel like drinking alcohol or even coffee. The sick cannot stomach junk food either, and so they might drink water or herbal tea and eat soups and salads, fruit and other light, digestible foods. They are listening to their bodies because they want to get better. It's as if all of a sudden, their taste buds have disappeared. They vow never to do wrong again, to start exercising and losing weight and have earlier nights. Of course, as soon as we feel better, all of our good intentions go out of the window, but a small seed has been planted.

> *"You don't need to change the world; you need to change yourself."*
>
> —*Miguel Rui*

When a person is not ready, progress will not happen. A person cannot be taught something they don't already know.

A person just reads or hears it differently, and when they are ready, the penny drops. In my work, when giving advice, I've encountered one of these situations: I either saw the light going on or I got a "but" in the response. Most of the time, though, people would find the answer in their own conversation. They just needed someone to talk to. So when the person had not done enough soul-searching, I heard many excuses in order for that person not to change. Oftentimes, the person would be right on the doorstep and need a little encouragement in order to go on and change. When it becomes obvious that change is going to happen (spiritual, emotional or physical), this feeling is one of uncertainty or fear. We must learn to welcome this and let life start teaching us her lessons. By this I mean it's a chance for us to do some soul-searching.

> "The real voyage of discovery consists not in seeking new landscapes, but in having new eyes."
>
> —Marcel Proust

We question our living situations, we look for answers, and we gradually become at ease with the change, and so progress has been made.

When life's lessons knock on our door and we ignore or resist the lesson, we become a *victim* of the situation, rather than *victorious*. Basically, when obstacles come into our lives, it's because we haven't learned that lesson yet. Since, in life, we must grow and learn, the same lesson will continue to knock on our door until we open up to it and change. We will always get an opportunity to learn from our mistakes. An example of this is the lure of stealing when we are young. Opportunity presents itself all around us: a chewy here, a lipstick there.

Some of us even get caught, and so we learn our lesson the hard way and never steal again, or the temptation will continue as opportunities continue all around us.

Here's an example: On a rainy day, a girl sitting next to you on the bus forgets her umbrella in the seat when she gets up at her stop, while you left yours at home. You are confronted with "two paths of opportunity." Which one will you take? Call out to the girl before she gets off the bus or look out of the window, waiting for the bus to safely drive on before clutching the umbrella in your own hands?

> "A man sooner or later discovers that he is the master-gardener of his soul, the director of his life."
> —James-Allen

For those who take the wrong path, similar situations of opportunity will happen again and again until we take the right path. For those who take the right path, we will feel triumph, and we instinctively know we made the right decision. Therefore, progress has occurred, and the wheel of life can continue in the right direction with the next new life lesson making its way to our door. We all have a choice to do right or wrong but the 'truth' does not give us a choice. Truth does not change.

> "The only way that we can live is if we grow. The only way that we can grow is if we change. The only way that we can change is if we learn. The only way we can learn is if we are exposed. And the only way that we can become exposed is if we throw ourselves out into the open. Do it. Throw yourself."
> —C. JoyBell C.

On this Earth, we all want the same thing: to love and to be loved; peace for all and regard for our fellow men. We would like to see kindness towards animals, and we would like to achieve environmental improvements of the Earth, since we borrowed it from our children. All these desires are on a level that connects us globally. It is within our society and social groups that we connect on an inner level. We share our feelings of hurt, jealousy, anger, contentment and happiness. Our communication with each other is so much better now. We can recommend books, websites and set up healing groups. We recognize those who need a helping hand, and it makes us feel good in return when we help to heal. We need to continue to heal others on a deeper, meaningful level. It is very important that we give of ourselves, whether it is through volunteer work, financial donations, emotional or spiritual support. We need to heal within, in order to heal the outside. That is when we can reduce suffering on every level.

> *"I slept and I dreamed that life is all joy. I woke and I saw that life is all service. I served and I saw that service is joy."*
> —*Kahlil Gibran*

So how does this relate to veganism? Well, as the wheels of life are turning, you will come across veganism one way or another. In the midst of our world, there will be moments when you are faced with it. You may feel it is not for you, and the lesson stops right there. Years may pass, and then you read an article on how many virgin forests are being destroyed in order to let a fast-food chain's cows graze on there. It might be water off a duck's back to you. That night, you watch a program on livestock being exported to the Middle East under horrific conditions, and it does make you think.

Perhaps it makes us think about our own suffering and death. Especially when we have a loved one who is dying, it makes us think about our own passing. People's perspective on life changes; meaning and purpose change. People look at their own missions in life. The death of a loved one changes our perspective. With this change, we relate to others differently. We act and think differently. We might even believe in something we once did not believe in. Change needs courage. You are a work in progress.

"Make a pact with yourself today to not be defined by your past. Sometimes the greatest thing to come out of all your hard work isn't what you get for it, but what you become for it. Shake things up today! Be You... Be Free... Share."
—Steve Maraboli

For the families of the terminally ill, this is a time for growth. For the person who is facing death, the experience is obviously even more life-changing. These people are forced to grow. They no longer need to work on the outer level but must look within on a spiritual level. They are stripped of their egos. Humility creeps in, as they are in God's hands. Many emotions will come up, feelings of guilt and the desire to make things right. In order to know what is going on within our emotional self, we need to be still. We need to meditate, listen to our soul, and this will lead to some level of awakening. These people have all the support of their family and friends. They will fit in with their loved one. The doctor tells the family not to give the patient red meat, in fact go vegan for a while; it is better for him. How often do we hear these people say they are thankful for their cancer? They are grateful for the experience of enlightenment. Some people even survive their cancer, and these people will never ever go back to the old ways, because they had a touch of enlightenment.

"If you would indeed behold the spirit of death,
open your heart wide into the body of life.
For life and death are one,
even as the river and the sea are one.

—*Kahlil Gibran*

Each and every one of us wants enlightenment, even if most of the 7 billion people on this planet don't realize it. We all seek love; we all want a better life ahead of us, compared to where we were before.

I wholeheartedly believe that with each awakening moment, we change for the better. Our outlook changes, our opinion changes, our diet changes and therefore our cells and our entire makeup changes. We no longer want to consume the blood of another. This vegan awakening will happen sooner or later. In my case, it was when I was six years old; in others, it may happen when they are sixty, and for many others, it will happen next time around. There is no correct sequence for this vegan awakening. I still have many lessons to learn; being a vegan was just one of the first on my path. I've known many wise people who still consume meat. Many people consume less and less and perhaps swap meat for fish. I do find generally that those who are the most awakened people of our time today are vegans, because a person who advocates kindness, selflessness and nonviolence could hardly be seen eating the flesh of another. I personally don't believe that our journey on this Earth is over unless you are a vegan, even if this is the last lesson we must learn. One cannot bring suffering to another, directly or indirectly; it's as simple as that!

Part Two

Nutrition and Veganism

I love the study of nutrition. I am very passionate about what it is within our foods that can heal us but also make us sick. I love studying cultures whose people lack sickness, have longevity, no crime and no doctors. All of this seems to be related. These cultures don't experience stress like we do. They seem to have an inborn happiness, a trust and a knowing which our society has lost generations ago. There is a healthy balance between spiritual, physical and emotional health, which each person practices. It is easy to see why our culture is in trouble. Stress is a killer of all three. Even though it may seem hopeless to try to have a balanced life, it isn't that hard. With a few changes, we can have a spiritually, physically and emotionally healthy life.

"Give freely to the world these gifts of love and compassion. Do not concern yourself with how much you receive in return, just know in your heart it will be returned."
—*Steve Maraboli,* Life, the Truth and Being Free

Soil

To me, it all starts with the soil our food grows in. If the soil is depleted nutritionally, there is no way the plant will grow healthy and strong. The plant will be weak and diseased. We must grow our food in natural, biochemically rich soil (soil rich in living organisms), sunlight, clean air and water. All plant life derives its nutrition this way. All other forms of life, including man, derive theirs from eating the plants or other living beings that eat these plants. Thus, humans cannot take in nutrients directly from the soil but need to eat the plants that grow in it in order to get the basic chemical elements to make us healthy. Therefore, when the soil lacks chemical elements, everything else moving up the food chain is affected.

Modern agriculture, determined to seek maximum harvest and profits, has changed the nature of the food we eat. We have strayed far away from a natural, pure and wholesome way of living. The food-processing industry has pushed the boundaries a lot further by providing us with a large selection of attractive, cheap, appealing and tasty substances that are totally insufficient in vitamins, enzymes, fibre and minerals.

> *"Man has only a thin layer of soil between himself and starvation."*
>
> *—Bart of Cincinnati*

Our bodies are not designed to ingest and assimilate these "foodless foods" or the additives that give these foods eternal shelf life in the supermarkets. When we eat these foodless foods, our systems are depleted nutritionally and become distressed from the toxins. Our tissues cannot be restored or rejuvenated without the proper foods. We need certain biochemical elements to restore health.

This is how it works: each organ and tissue type needs certain different kinds of chemical elements to do its job properly in the overall functioning of the body. Our bones and teeth are primarily calcium and phosphorus in structure. The chemical element of skin and hair is mostly silicon, so even though it is made up of keratin, its chemical element which keeps keratin healthy is silicon. Silicon also makes our muscles firmer. Iron is an element important in the blood. Since every organ, tissue and microscopic cell contributes to the well-being of the body, it is very important, whether our food's chemicals are deficient or not. Without ample biochemicals in our soil and therefore our food and bodies, wellness cannot be achieved and sustained, no matter what we do.

> "The best six doctors anywhere
> And no one can deny it
> Are sunshine, water, rest, and air
> exercise and diet.
> These six will gladly you attend
> If only you are willing
> Your mind they'll ease
> Your will they'll mend
> And charge you not a shilling.
> —Nursery rhyme quoted by Wayne Fields,
> What the River Knows, 1990

The Alkaline and Acidic Diet

This is not some "new age" diet; it has been around for a very long time. The founder of its name was William Hay, who originally called it the Acidic/Alkaline and Neutral Diet back in 1920. He was an admirer of Hippocrates, the father of medicine and the one who laid down the foundations of a healthy diet. Hippocrates said, "Food should be our medicine and our medicine should be our food." This was back in 431 BC. Yes, 431 BC! Hippocrates believed in raw food, especially green-leafed food. He did not include meats, cheese, or milk in the diet when a person needed to be healed. He knew the importance of elimination and always looked at the whole person when curing him, such as what external influences could have contributed to the ill health, like stress, climate, dampness in the house, as well as an unbalanced and deficient nutritional diet.

> "A patient cured is a customer lost."
>
> —William Hay

The rules are very simple. The circles represent our daily food.

Alkaline / Acidic balance

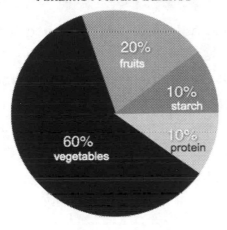

80% of our daily diet should be alkaline with 20% being alkaline fruits and 60% being vegetables

20% of our daily diet should be acidic with 10% being starch and 10% being protein

Raw / Cooked balance

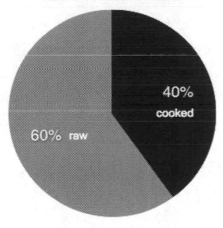

60% of our daily diet should be raw

40% of our daily diet should be cooked

Food should be cooked as little as possible, not microwaved, boiled or deep fried.

> *"For the best health, a body should be at the very least slightly alkaline at 7.35 to 7.45 pH."*
>
> —*Dr. Bernard Jensen*

This breaks down to eating at least six different veggies, two alkaline fruits, one starch and one protein every day. Do not have starch and protein in the same meal. Have each one separately with veggies. Most alkaline food, once it is cooked, will turn acidic and has very little nutrition left in it. I feel fruit should be eaten by itself during snack time or first thing in the morning. If you follow this diet, you will have more energy, you won't feel bloated, you'll lose weight, and your immunity will strengthen.

Why is alkalinity so important in our diet? All disease conditions originally begin with a chemical deficiency or with too many toxins in a person's body. Look at it this way: the moment we die, our body becomes very acidic, in order to start the decomposition process. So, if we toxify our bodies, they *will* become acidic. Basically, our body starts to break down as it would if we were dead, resulting in arthritis, osteoporosis, stiffness, loss of good sight and hearing, and chronic fatigue and aging. Our veins and arteries, our regulatory systems, our organs and our hormone systems are all interfered with. This is what happens! We ferment from the inside out.

All deaths are the endpoint of progressive acid saturation. Eat acidity, and you'll give your body the go-ahead to break down. We become old because there is too much acidity in our systems. When we become acidic, blood cannot flow freely because our capillaries become thinner and therefore clump the blood together. Our blood has a pH of 7.4.

Did you know that we cannot survive long if our pH goes below 7.2? This is because our blood cannot carry oxygen. People with chronic fatigue syndrome have a blood pH of 7.2. In this state, we have lower levels of oxygen and energy. This lowers our immune system, and all this because we consume too many acidic foods and drinks.

The only way back to health is to eat and drink alkaline food and drinks. A strong immune system will fight off viruses and bacteria, and it can deal with a bit of toxicity every now and then.

> *"Acid food leads to pain, disease and death, while alkalinity leads to better health and longevity."*
> *—Sang Whang 2002 Sang Whang Enterprises.*

The health of our body is determined by the health of each cell. A healthy cell is alkaline, and a cancer cell is acidic. Our body constantly fights to maintain an alkaline blood pH. One way is to pull stored sodium, calcium and magnesium from our bones and teeth to neutralize blood acids. This is why we have arthritis and stiffness targeting the outer parts of our body, to keep toxins away for as long as possible from our vital organs like the heart and lungs. What we eat and drink has a direct result on our blood-pH levels. I highly recommend looking up alkaline diets on the Internet. There is an alkaline cookbook called *The Alkaline Diet Recipe Book.*

For those people who are overweight, the culprit is always acidic food. Even if you want to lose as little as two kilograms, all you have to do is cut out acidic food. You don't need to diet. You can eat as much alkaline food as you like. I'm even going as far as to say that you don't need to include exercise in this case—even though I am a big believer in exercise. All I am saying is, if you do exercise and you still have problems losing weight, then you don't need to increase your exercise; just cut out acidic food. Your metabolism will get faster and stronger. You'll become more flexible, thinner; your skin will look better; bags under the eyes will lessen and getting up in the morning will be easier.

We are what we eat, or, more specifically, we are what we absorb. Those beautiful cakes we pop into our mouths are eventually responsible for developing every cell in our bodies and affect not only our physical health but also the way we think. Negativity and stress destroy vital chemicals.

For example, stress and worry acidify the body and ultimately cause ulcers. Fatigue can be caused by bitterness, unforgiveness and worry. Thyroid imbalance is due to emotional hurt and sadness. Glandular problems are due to fear. Louise Hay wrote many books on this subject, such as *You Can Heal Your Life.* I am sure that many of you are familiar with this book, and if not, it is a good one to have. It basically explains the correlation between our thinking and the physical problems we have.

"My body is a glorious place to live. It serves me so well. I choose the healing thoughts that create and maintain my healthy body and make me feel good. I love and appreciate my beautiful body."

—Louise L. Hay

Chemical Elements[1]

We have many different biochemical elements in our bodies that are necessary for proper health. Unhealthy foods and a negative mental attitude deplete our chemical reserves, resulting in disease. I find that the most important chemical elements are calcium, iodine, sodium and silicon. There are many more, but these are the ones that are so often depleted. There are sixteen biochemical elements we need for our health and well-being. They are: calcium, iodine, sodium, silicon, magnesium, potassium, iron, sulphur, oxygen, carbon, hydrogen, nitrogen, phosphorus, chlorine, fluorine and manganese. There are many more trace elements which are also of extreme importance. All elements are found in a large variety of foods. Therefore, we need to eat these foods regularly and over a large period of time, as it feeds every cell in the body, making it healthy, physically and emotionally.

Calcium—"The Knitter": Calcium is stored in the bones, and calcium is the knitter. This chemical element is needed in every organ of the body, even in the brain. Calcium gives us courage and the power to carry through. It makes the will stronger and builds strength and endurance. The greatest enemy of calcium is sugar because it leaches calcium from the body...

> *"In order to change, we must be sick and tired of being sick and tired."*
>
> *—Author Unknown*

There is calcium in seeds, the outer leaves of cabbage, kale, spinach, cranberries, tahini, avocados, broccoli, carrots, lentils, dulse, kelp and any green organic juices.

Iodine—"The Metaboliser": When our bodily functions become underactive, we must look at the thyroid gland. It needs iodine through foods. Dulse and dulse tablets are great. Calcium is also needed when iodine levels are low. A thyroid breaks down when a person breaks down emotionally.

Similarly, ulcers are caused by work stress. No amount of iodine is going to fix an unhappy and sad heart. We need to change emotionally as well. Foods high in iodine include kelp and dulse, okra, agar, asparagus, beans, blueberries, carrots, cucumber, coconuts, kale, seaweed, strawberries, tofu, watercress, papayas, mangoes, pineapples and watermelon *with* the seeds.

> *"The role of calcium in the body is similar to that in the soil. It aids digestion, nutrition and neutralization, promotes good growth, solidity and vigor by helping to regulate metabolism properly."*
>
> *—Dr. Bernard Jensen*

Sodium—"The Youth Element": Sodium is stored in the stomach, joints and digestive system. Please note: Table-salt is *not* sodium. Table-salt is a drug and a preservative. It is not a food and should not be consumed. Sodium makes calcium and magnesium more soluble and convertible into bone tissue. Sodium is stored in the joints and gastrointestinal system walls. When our body becomes depleted of sodium, then our joints pick up calcium deposits, the stomach becomes acidic and bowel elimination becomes underactive. Sodium is stored in the stomach walls first and in the joints secondly, so whenever we find joint trouble, there is stomach trouble. For example, heartburn indicates a need for sodium, and therefore a diet of celery and okra is a high priority. For good health, along with the joints, stomach and lungs, the lymph glands must be in good order as well. In them we find a sodium reserve, and a good sodium reserve is essential in order to get well and stay well. Arthritis is a nutritional-deficiency disease. It means that calcium has come out of solution in the blood and deposits in the joints.

> "Arthritis is a nutritional deficiency disease. If we all eat the nutrients we need, we can live out our lives without the misery of arthritis."
>
> —Dr. Ruth Yale Long

Sodium and vitamin C are needed to bring calcium back to solution. Of course, by vitamin C, I mean *natural* vitamin C, found in food like kiwifruit and home-grown, organic, sun-ripened oranges picked from the tree and eaten straight away. It is also found in melons, berries, apples, spinach, home-grown strawberries, celery and parsley. Vitamin C is destroyed by heat, air and light. Vitamin C is not stored in the body and must be replaced every day.

Vitamin C pills are useless, as it does not get absorbed by the body. Most vegetables and fruit possess an organic, biochemical form of sodium, compatible with the human body. Table salt and chemical salts contain inorganic sodium, which is not at all compatible with the human body. Children who lack sodium are prone to be sick. Sodium is highly alkaline and therefore named the "youth element," by Dr Bernard Jensen, as it promotes youthfulness, with flexible joints. Foods high in sodium are raw, organic, fresh goat's milk; apples; apricots; asparagus; celery; kale; kelp; okra; parsley; spinach; sesame and sunflower seeds.

> *"With lentils, tomatoes and rice, olives and nuts and bread,*
> *Why does a man care to gnaw a slice of something bleeding*
> *and dead?"*
>
> *—Henry Bailey Stevens*

Silicon—"The Tough Element": Silicon is stored in the hair, nails and skin. Silicon gives firmness to stalks of grains and produces a polished, hard outer layer on oats, barley, rice and corn. Silicon is found in the outer shell of seeds and nuts and the outer peeling of fruits and vegetables. The highest concentration is in the rice peeling. That is why you must always have brown rice, never white. It also gives hardness, firmness, elasticity and polish to teeth and toughness to tendons and bones. Silicon supports the outer lining of many foods; similarly, it protects the outer lining of beings. Nails, hair and skin derive their health from silicon. Oat-straw tea is very high in silicon, as is shavegrass and flaxseed tea and alfalfa. Other foods high in silicon are: apples, apricots, asparagus, bananas, barley, beans, beetroot, carrots, cauliflower, celery, corn, kelp, nectarines, oats, pumpkin, brown and wild rice, spinach, sprouted seeds, sweet potatoes and sunflower seeds.

> *"Negative passions such as hatred, outbursts, jealousy,*
> *quarrels, resentment, bitterness, hostility, selfishness and*
> *greed use up magnesium."*
>
> *—Dr. Bernard Jensen*

Magnesium—"The Relaxer": Magnesium is widely available in foods, but very little of it is absorbed, digested and assimilated. Magnesium deficiency shows when a person is constipated and often manifests as sleeplessness. When someone has a magnesium deficiency, the nervous system becomes hyperactive; this means that the person is highly emotionally charged. Magnesium is necessary to calm nerves and clean the digestive tract. Magnesium makes our muscles more flexible and is highly alkaline. In addition to this, it gives us restful sleep, as it combats acids, toxins and gasses and therefore purifies the body.

We find that yellow foods are the highest in magnesium. All yellow foods have laxative elements in them. These foods include yellow squash, corn, apricots and yellow cornmeal. When a person is constipated reach out to yellow foods. Make corn soup or eat corn, fruits and salads. What we should not do is reach for a laxative drug that is not derived from food. It irritates the bowels, and that is why we go, because our body wants to expel it. Even worse is to reach out for a cigarette and a cup of coffee in order to relax. Coffee has been proven to cause dehydration and rectal cancer; it is coffee that makes us constipated in the first place.

> "If you want to lift yourself up, lift up someone else."
> —Booker T. Washington

Coffee, sugar, smoking and alcohol have disastrous impact on our magnesium metabolism. We also need to work on our attitudes to reduce tension. Magnesium will assist us in soothing the nerves, but we need calmness in our hearts, in order to keep reserves up. Other foods high in magnesium are avocados, bananas, nuts, okra, parsley, tofu, endive, lentils and beetroot.

Potassium—"The Great Alkaliser": Nearly all people are in need of potassium, which is an alkaliser for the body. Potassium assists the recuperative powers to restore the rich alkaline salts to the blood. Potassium and sodium (not salt) work together in all cells of the body, neutralising acids.

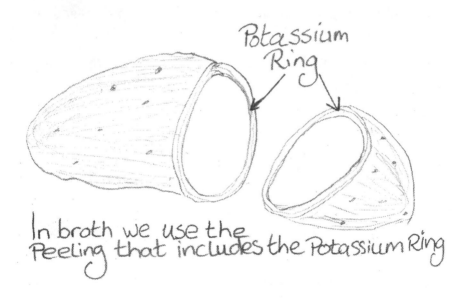

Potassium Ring

In broth we use the peeling that includes the Potassium Ring

> "All green tops of vegetables are high in potassium. Potassium is the bitter elements in foods, whereas sodium is the sweet element in foods."
>
> —Dr. Bernard Jensen

If you suffer rheumatic or arthritic conditions, you need potassium so that acids can leave the joints. Potassium increases alkalinity and reduces acidity. Potato-peeling broth is excellent for getting potassium. Take three large, organic, ripe potatoes, and cut the peeling at least a half centimetre thick. Throw the centre of the potato away, because this is the acidic part of the potato. Use four organic carrots, eight sticks of celery, and a handful of parsley. Cut this all up and put it in a pot and cover with water. Do not boil, but keep the heat semi-high for fifteen minutes. Strain off and drink the liquid. Do this for thirty days.

Eat alkaline, raw salads, and after only three days, you'll feel the difference. Any pain due to stiffness and arthritis would have a chance to leave the body. We find potassium in the tops of vegetables like celery and watercress. A teaspoon of organic apple-cider vinegar in warm water first thing in the morning is also very high in potassium. Other high-potassium foods are: bananas, figs, organic raw sun-ripened tomatoes, apples, almonds, most beans, beetroot, blackberries and blueberries, broccoli, carrots, cucumbers, dulse, dates, grapes with seeds, kelp, parsley, sage tea, tahini, soymilk, spinach, watercress, the green outer leaves of lettuce (not the lighter green; this is too acidic to have any nutritional value) and alfalfa sprouts.

Iron—"The Frisky Horse Element": Iron is our blood builder, but it needs oxygen as well. Oxygen is the giver of life. Iron is stored in every organ of the body but particularly in the liver. One-fourth of our blood is in the liver at any one time being purified, but it needs oxygen to burn up the toxic wastes. Oxygen provides the warmth needed for elimination. Iron must evolve through plants, which are organic, in order for us to absorb the iron. Inorganic iron is useless to us. We need the vitamin C in foods in order for iron to be absorbed. Inorganic iron, like the kind your doctor prescribes when your iron levels are low, is rapidly rejected and expelled by the body through the kidneys and bowel. This is why you get constipated when you take these tablets. Your iron levels will improve on paper, but the iron is not used in the right way. You will still feel tired. There is no vitamin C in them, and vitamin C is a natural laxative. The highest-iron foods also have very high vitamin C, like blackberries. Also, deep breathing and exercise will help the oxygen levels in your body, which also helps to absorb iron. Iron and oxygen fit like a hand in a glove; one cannot be considered without the other.

> *"Inorganic iron is valuable to the pharmaceutical companies but disastrous to the body."*
>
> *—Dr. Bernard Jensen*

Iron is more readily assimilated from fruits and vegetables juices than from solid cooked food. The average person's diet is deficient in iron because iron is not high in many foods. Even foods high in iron like spinach, if grown in iron-poor soil, will be lacking high iron levels. All iron-bearing foods should be eaten raw or juiced. Never soak or boil these foods, because it destroys the iron. If you must cook it, steam it for a very short time. This causes at least 46 percent iron loss, so drink the liquid. One of the best iron sources is liquid chlorophyll. Chlorophyll is the green colour in plant life. You can purchase liquid chlorophyll from any health-food shop or maybe even the health section in your supermarket. Nature's Sunshine has a lovely-tasting one, and I recommend a squirt in a glass of water every time. Get your children used to it. Yes, the colour is green, but so is green cordial. It is a great cleanser for the body.

Other iron-rich foods include: black cherries, organic molasses, dulse, greens, fennel, kelp, lentils, parsley, pumpkin seeds, radishes, rice polishings, walnuts, tahini, tofu, tempeh, sprouted seeds, sunflower seeds, soybeans and dried beans which you put in your soups and stews.

Interestingly, in the top fifty-five foods highest in iron there was not even a mention of meat or any other meat products. In fact, there was not even a mention of meat in any of the research done on iron, even though the researchers were pro-meat. Page 217, The Chemistry of Man, Dr Bernard Jensen. This is because even though meat is high in iron, it does not contain any vitamin C and therefore cannot be absorbed by the body. In addition, we need to cook the meat, which destroys iron anyway.

Vegans do not have to have lower iron levels than meat-eaters. In fact, the absorption of iron is much higher in vegans than in meat-eaters because of the high vitamin C content vegans eat in their regular diet. Also, calcium, coffee and tea reduce iron absorption. Iron deficiency is the most common nutritional disorder in the western world, yet 95 percent of these people eat meat. New studies on iron absorption are happening all the time, and the data your doctor has may be out of date. If you want to learn more, you can read a very informative paper online written by Elizabeth C. Theil and Jean- Francois Briat called *Plant Ferritin and Non-Heme Iron Nutrition in Humans.*

> *"Whole foods like grains and beans release their sugar very, very slowly because of the fiber in them, and they don't give you a sugar rush. They feed your cells as needed, and as a result, you have loads of stable energy that powers you through the day."*
>
> —*Kathy Freston*

Sulphur—"The Heating Element": This lively element drives impurities to the surface of the skin and produces heat within the body. Along with phosphorus and manganese, sulphur is a brain and nerve element. It drives nutrition to the brain. We must therefore include sulphur vegetables in our diet. Sulphur foods help promote the flow of bile, aid elimination and stimulate cells. Sulphur vegetables are also known as winter vegetables, because they can withstand the cold weather. Sulphur also forces lecithin to the brain and nervous system, which is very important. It is hard to get any lecithin to our brains, so sulphur foods are very important to us. They do produce gas, especially when eaten raw, but if our system is strong enough, it will digest properly. Lightly steaming is best for these vegetables. Please be careful with sulphur-treated fruit. Dried foods like sultanas are often treated with sulphur which is a chemical and can bring on serious illnesses.

> *"Redheads get the color of their hair from sulphur and their familiar temperaments are largely a result of the sulphur in their body chemistry."*
>
> —*Dr. Bernard Jensen*

When eaten in a normal supply through vegetables, this element will promote youth and beauty. Sulphur cleans and heats the blood. The highest-sulphur foods include: kale, cabbage, brussels sprouts, cauliflower, watercress, chervil, horseradish, cranberries, broccoli and onions.

Oxygen—"The Giver of Life": Whenever we have a lot of oxygen in the body, all faculties improve. We feel better when we exercise and breathe in fresh air. Life demands heat, and heat demands oxygen. The brain requires more than four times as much oxygen as the rest of the body to repair and build tissues. Your metabolism is strengthened by oxygen. Overweight and unhealthy people lack oxygen. We need oxygen when we need to rebuild ourselves. Yawning is often a sign that the brain needs oxygen. For oxygen to work properly in our bodies, we need sunlight on our bodies, deep breathing, and foods high in oxygen, iron, potassium, sulphur and phosphorus.

Vegetables and fruits in their raw state are high-oxygen foods. Even juiced, they are still highly beneficial for us. A diet high in protein, carbohydrates, starches, sugars, fats, sulphur and heavy meals in general lower oxidation in the body. Alive, raw foods include rainbow salads, fruit salads, raw-food platters and sprouts. Other foods include: nuts and seeds, beetroot, blueberries, carrots, figs, grapes, capsicum, leeks, spinach, and organically grown and ripened tomatoes.

Carbon—"The Builder": Carbon in food form occurs mainly in sugar, starch, sweets, fats and most proteins. When there is too much carbon in a person's system, it leads to obesity. Almost all people eat too many carbohydrates. It makes us want to sit or lie down. All sugary and starchy foods lead to too much carbon. We need carbon to build all integral functions, but a balance is necessary here. The best foods to support this building element are: lentil casserole, rice polishings, barley, nut butters, avocados, almonds, olive and peanut oils, popcorn, apricots, apples, beans, buckwheat, corn, dates, figs, oats, pears, peas, prunes, rye and wheat bran.

> *"Muscle metabolism highly depends on carbon, as muscles demand sugar for warmth and energy."*
> —*Dr. Bernard Jensen*

Hydrogen—"The Moisturizer": Hydrogen is essential for the progression of digestion, nutrition assimilation, and elimination. It is vital for transporting nutrients through the arteries to the brain and tissues of all the parts of the body. It also aids in the regulation of body temperature. Hydrogen prevents inflammation, as it soothes the nerves. Although water, which is actually a food, is only 11 percent hydrogen, certain foods like pears are 83 percent water (9 percent hydrogen); watermelon is 93 percent water.

People who hold water in their system have too much sodium and not enough potassium. I find this element very important, as it is the moisturizer of all vegetable, animal and human life. High-hydrogen foods are high in water like apricots, asparagus, blackberries and blueberries, broccoli, carrots, celery, cherries, guavas, mangos, okra, papayas, parsley, peaches, pineapple, prunes, pumpkin, radishes, sauerkraut, sorrel, spinach, strawberries, organic sun-ripened tomatoes, watercress and watermelon. Citrus fruits contain a lot of water, but I would only recommend eating them if they have been sun-ripened and eaten as soon as you've picked them from the tree. Do not eat citrus out of season. Fresh fruit and vegetable juices (the ones you make yourself) are also very high-hydrogen liquids. Do not mix the two. Just have vegetable juice like carrots, celery and cucumber or fruit juice like pineapple, papaya and mango juice. Watermelon juice should be drunk (and eaten) by itself.

Nitrogen—"The Restrainer": Nitrogen is part of each protein, to some degree; whether it is in plants, animals or man, it is in food and in the air. Nitrogen, in conjunction with the three vital elements—hydrogen, carbon and oxygen—is important for power and vigour of all organisms, as it is a tissue-builder. Nitrogen is essential for our metabolism to be complete. It is a restraining element, the opposite of oxygen.

Oxygen is like fire, whereas nitrogen is stillness itself. People who are fatigued and absentminded need more nitrogen in their systems. Legumes store nitrogen in the nodules on their roots, which they have taken from the air. If the roots are allowed to remain in the soil and be composted, the nitrogen is therefore released into the soil. This process greatly enriches the soil, as it adds to its vitality. This process is called "green manuring" when the plants are ploughed back into the soil. Foods highest in nitrogen are beans (dried and fresh), black-eyed peas, butternut pumpkin, nuts and spinach, lentils and leafy greens.

"Nitrogen foods are high-protein foods. It is not advisable that one consumes animal protein as a nitrogen food, as it quickly becomes in excess, having a very negative result in our system as it acidifies, and wounds refuse to heal."
—Dr. Bernard Jensen

Phosphorus—"The Light Bearer": Phosphorus improves the nutrition of the nervous system. Bones are made denser, and the reproductive organs are favourably affected when phosphorus is supplied in proper quantities. This element is a nerve and brain tonic; with each thought, phosphorus is used up. Phosphorus must undergo transformations, beginning in mineral form, moving from there to the soil by decay, and then into seeds and grains and ultimately into the human brain.

Children at school or anyone studying must have brain phosphorus in their daily diet. If nutrition is poor, the blood cannot nourish the brain. Phosphorus also comes from the animal kingdom, and this might tip the balance too much towards this element. If there is too much phosphorus in the brain, the person becomes delusional. This delusion encourages the feeling of false pride, and he will preach to others, as he feels he is the chosen one. They will arrogantly dictate that they know all, even when they are wrong and know very little. Also, phosphorus from the animal kingdom is high in cholesterol, acidity and fats, therefore better left alone.

"Without phosphorus, we could not study, memorize, read, reason, create, visualize and comprehend. Each activity of the brain and nerve cell requires phosphorus."
—Dr. Bernard Jensen

Oxygen is important for recovery. Phosphorus is found in almost every food: rice and oat bran, barley, beans (fresh and dried), cabbage, carrots, nuts, corn, dulse, kelp, lentils, millet, pumpkin seeds, rye, seeds, walnuts, tempeh, tahini, soybean and flaxseed. Alcohol reduces phosphorus levels, as does salt and medication.

> "Getting well may be a matter of educating rather than medicating."
>
> —Dr. Bernard Jensen

Chlorine: "The Cleanser": Chlorine made in a factory is a killer for our health, but it is the most wonderful element when we find it in our foods, as it cleanses and rejuvenates. Chlorine is an element that gets rid of waste matter, cleanses the blood and keeps joints and tendons supple. Chlorine is the best element for ending stomach troubles by helping the hydrochloric acid become balanced again, which in turn gets rid of gas in the body. Chlorine found in celery and its juice, along with carrots and their juice, is perhaps our greatest cleanser. It is found in all greens and salad vegetables and fruits. If it weren't for chlorine in foods, we would not have a clean body.

Other foods high in chlorine include: asparagus, avocados, bananas, beans, beetroot, coconut, corn, cucumbers, dandelion greens, eggplant, endive, guava, kale, kelp, leeks, lentils, dark-green leaves of lettuce, mangos, peaches, pineapples, potatoes with skins, radishes, raspberries, spinach, seeds, sweet potatoes, watercress and watermelon.

Fluorine—"The Anti-Resistant Element": Fluorine is very important today because so much food is cooked, treated, canned and packaged, therefore destroying this element.

It is only available to us in raw food, and 60 percent of our food should be raw. In a sense, fluorine is a beauty and youth element when provided in ample quantities in the diet.

In conjunction with calcium, it forms strong bones, tough tooth enamel and healthy hair and nails. We only need the tiniest amount in our system for it to work sufficiently. It works as a disinfectant and an antiseptic and is effective against fever, toxins and acids. Fluorine improves absorption of magnesium phosphate, sodium chloride and calcium carbonate, as long as it is supplied in the organic form. The spleen must have fluorine in order to function properly, otherwise it will become enlarged. Aching eyeballs or any discharge coming from the eyes is also an indication of fluorine starvation. The difference between fluorine and fluoride is that fluorine is an element which cannot be broken down, and fluoride is a compound which has fluorine in it. Foods high in fluorine are: avocados, black-eyed peas, brussels sprouts, cabbage, cauliflower, dates, endive, greens, lemongrass, licorice (the real stuff), spinach, parsley, rice, and organic sun-ripened tomatoes.

We need only the smallest amount of fluorine. Adding it to water and toothpaste is not safe, and there is growing concern about the health damage it is doing to people. Never give it to children. Have fluorine only in its organic state.
—Dr Bernard Jensen.

Manganese—"The Love Element": Manganese is called the "love element" because when we have it in our bodies, we can show unconditional love and more patience and relate better to those around us. Manganese is found in the linings of the brain and the heart. It is found in the bloodstream, and its metabolism is similar to that of iron. Iron-rich foods are also good sources of manganese.

> *Any catarrhal condition is caused by catarrhal-producing foods. Immunity is weakened because of these foods, and so the only way for us to get rid of catarrh is to get sick and throw it all out. The worst thing we can do is to stop this cleaning-out process. We should support it by rosting, eating light, digestible foods, and increase our vitamin C intake.*
> *—Sandra Kimler*

People are susceptible to absent-mindedness when they are lacking manganese. They are impatient, and depression lingers. A person so tired that she cannot stand up straight is lacking manganese and calcium. As with all other elements, it must be supplied to our bodies in organic form, evolved biochemically from the soil. Foods high in manganese include: walnuts, seeds, apples, apricots, beans, blackberries and blueberries, butternut pumpkin, cardamom, celery, chestnuts, dark-green vegetable leaves, mint, oats, parsley, pineapples, rye and watercress.

So there you have it, our sixteen vital biochemical elements which are needed for our well-being. Many foods have lots of the different elements in them, and others are severely lacking in the variety of elements. For example: nuts are low in chlorine but have the other fifteen elements in them. Bread is deficient in nine of the sixteen elements. Honey is very low in fourteen of the sixteen elements and is extremely high in sugar. Raw potatoes are low in five elements, but when boiled, they are almost entirely water and starch. Kale is extremely high in three of the elements (calcium, sodium and iodine) but is low in four. As you can see, it is because of this that we need a large variety of fresh food to get all the chemical elements to make us shine inside and out! It also shows the correlation between our behaviour and the elements. Our behaviour is very much affected by the lack of chemical elements in our body. Therefore, when we say you need a good balance of *all* sixteen elements for health, we include our emotional welfare in that as well as our physical health.

> "Our demand for meat, dairy and refined carbohydrates—the world consumes one billion cans or bottles of Coke a day—our demand for these things, not our need, our want—drives us to consume way more calories than are good for us."
>
> —Mark Bittman

This former information might have been a little boring for you, but I included it because it shows how important live foods are. It also shows how important live soils are. Depleted soils mean depleted chemical elements in our food, resulting in an imbalance in our bodies, resulting in dis-ease. You can also see that the same element is present in a variety of foods. I gave you only a small example of which foods contain which elements. We need to eat alive foods all the time like all the different sprouts, all the different nuts, all the beans, all the fruit that is in season, all the vegetables that are in season, legumes and seeds.

Health, then, is restored by getting rid of toxins, by eating food with the right chemical elements and by changing to positive attitudes and emotional patterns. It is therefore of the utmost importance that we eat a variety of foods and also include all the colours of the rainbow. Health diminishes when deficiencies in the chemistry in our system occur. A healthy person has a balance of all the elements working in harmony with each other, as well as a happy outlook on life. The approach of Western medicine is all geared to stop the symptom.

"We all love animals. Why do we call some 'pets' and others 'dinner'?"

—k.d. lang

Next time you go to the doctor, ask where the source of your ailment came from. He or she will have no idea. At best, the doctor will guess. Then you should ask, "Is there any food I should eat to make this better?" This is when you'll get a puzzled, perplexed look on your doctor's face, saying, "No, no, food has nothing to do with it." Try it; it really works. It is not the doctors' fault; they do not study nutrition. They can study, if they want to, a little course in dietary studies, where they will become familiar with the Food Pyramid. They will prescribe antibiotics, and you will be on your merry way, costing this country millions! Did you know that 22 million prescriptions are filled out here in Australia every year? Well, now you do. I believe that almost all of these are unnecessary.

Acidity causes the start of all discomforts, diseases and weaknesses. Do you realize that you, *YES, you* have so much more power over your health than your doctor? You have so much more power over your body. Don't panic too quickly. Sickness is a way for your body to throw out toxins. It is a way for your body to get a rest from the foods you normally eat. The flu, sore throats, earaches, bronchitis, headaches, tummy upsets, allergies, constipation, diarrhoea, runny noses, and boils that won't go away are all results of us eating the wrong foods for too long and way too much.

> *"A man of my spiritual intensity does not eat corpses."*
> —George Bernard Shaw

Iridology

I used to foster children, and the first thing I'd do when they came to live with me was to change their diet. That wasn't easy, as all the children were used to sugary, fatty foods and soft drinks. Some never even had raw, green food, and drinking plain water was unheard of. The first thing was to give them liquid chlorophyll to drink; absolutely no junk food. I would not even give them heavy foods like potatoes, white rice and bread. Why not bread? Well, what do you put on bread? It is either sweet or salty; not good for cleaning out a body's system. I gave them lots of raw greens and fruit.

I did give them wraps with grated beetroot, carrots, dark lettuce leaves, cucumber, sprouts and a sprinkle of mixed herbs, but no salt or sauces. The first three days were always a challenge, because these children were withdrawing from the sugar, salt and fats. I made sure they had these foods to snack on all day, talked to them a lot, and just tried to take their minds off the fact that they didn't have a packet of chips in one hand and a Coke bottle in the other.

After three days, these children became far more manageable, pleasant and kind. The older children even started to help with the dishes and help around the house. They also went back to school and even did their homework without too much fuss. The babies I had in my foster-care all came with snotty noses; they were not sleeping, unsettled and often crying. They also came with cow's-milk formula. I changed this to soy formula, which is far more compatible with a baby's digestive system. I also gave them lukewarm water with chlorophyll, which they seemed to enjoy. These babies took no time at all to settle down. After their first drink of soy milk, they often slept peacefully. The red, pimply skin disappeared within two days, along with the snotty noses. Stools improved and smelled less, and I ended up with gorgeous, happy babies who were not hard to handle at all (usually the reason they were put into my care in the first place).

Being an iridologist, the interest for me was the change in the colour of the children's eyes. I noticed that the children's eyes changed quickly. They went from murky green or hazel to deep blue. Those with light-blue eyes also turned deep blue. Healing lines appeared right through the eyes, showing how quickly our bodies can reverse the damage that was caused by the wrong foods.

"Because the eye and iris are composed of all major tissues of the body, iridology as a science of the eye, is useful in assessing the body's physiology healing signs as a person improves lifestyle and his mental/emotional/ spiritual habits."

—Dr. Bernard Jensen

Iridology is the science of interpreting tissue conditions from the iris of the eye, revealing through structure, colour and markings which organs and tissues are chemically depleted.

This is shown by dark areas or very light acidic areas, and as your diet improves, the dark area in your iris will get light healing lines. It is a very easy science to grasp. The whole body appears in the iris, which is viewed as a clock face; 12:00 is our head area, and as the hand of the clock goes down, so do our body parts. Our middle part at 3:00 and 6:00 represents our legs and feet. As we go back up to 9:00, it represents our organs and back area of our body.

Our irises do mirror each other. The chart on the next page will give you an indication of what I am talking about. There is no hocus-pocus here. This is a very precise science. I find it such a pity that doctors of Western medicine don't study iridology. I'll give you an example: A child grows up diagnosed with asthma, has all the medications including the puffers she needs, and is hospitalized many times because of its severity. Then in her late teens, she goes to an iridologist, who reveals that her back is out, causing an improper blood supply to the bronchial area. This area has become laden with toxins, which has caused asthma. So this person then goes and has her back aligned, which was out because of an old injury when she fell off a swing at five years old. The blood supply is returned in full to the upper body area, and toxins are moved along; therefore, no more asthma. That girl was me, and I never had an asthma attack again. The iridologist also told me to stop eating dairy products, to help the elimination process.

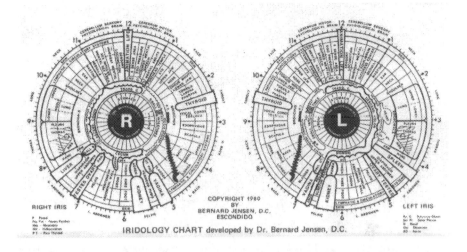

IRIDOLOGY CHART developed by Dr. Bernard Jensen, D.C.

"Most people are very mobile and do not follow a sufficiently powerful rejuvenation program to achieve... results. But for those who are really making progress in healing, the iris changes are evident."

—Dr. Bernard Jensen

If my doctor had studied iridology, then he would have picked up my back injury instantly, preventing years of asthma attacks and medication. Of course, most times, asthma is caused by dairy products, but that also can be picked up in iridology.

I will share with you how I came to study iridology. It was in my late teens that a Pap smear came back positive for abnormal cells. So I had the standard laparoscopy and burning away of the abnormal cells. After ten days, I had another test done, and the abnormal cells were back. My mother decided then that she would take me to see Dr. Bernard Jensen in California. She had started to study nutrition and felt he might have a better solution to this problem.

We went to his Health Ranch in Escondido. There he revealed through iridology that I had a leaky lower bowel, which caused the abnormal cells, and it was not cervical cancer. He immediately changed my diet. No more junk food. (I ate Chiko Rolls every day.) I had to clean out my system, and I did a seven-day cleanse which included two colemas a day. When we returned, I had another Pap smear, and my results were negative. The doctor asked what happened, but when I told him I had done a cleanse and changed my diet, he shrugged it off. My doctor had no interest; in fact, he said that diet had no relevance to my becoming better. This was thirty years ago, and luckily, doctors are now far more aware that diet has a huge influence on our health.

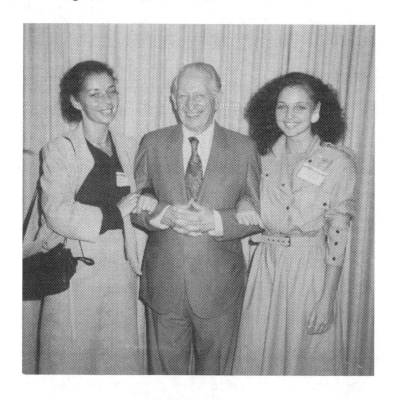

From left to right: My beautiful mum, Hennie Spykers-Hersman, Dr. Bernard Jensen and me.

> *"A highly sensitive person can eat the healthiest possible food and still experience a breakdown of health in a nerve-wracking urban environment. An ambitious, talented person may live in a quiet, slow-moving rural area, eat nutritious food and still experience loss of health from the lack of challenge in life."*
>
> *—Dr. Bernard Jensen*

It was after this trip to California that my mum and eventually I myself started studying nutritional diet and lifestyle seriously. We attended many of Dr. Bernard Jensen's lectures and seminars and even went to his eightieth birthday party. Even though he has passed away, I am still his student, and I am very grateful that my mum took me to see him.

> *"I personally believe that temperaments, foods, types, culture, altitude, environment, inheritance, living habits and sunshine all go together to make the man."*
>
> *—Dr. Bernard Jensen*

My research into health continues, and I wish doctors would take this outlook more seriously. Doctors are aware that the wrong food causes diabetes and heart disease, but unfortunately, they tend to study the Food Pyramid, which includes foods we should not consume in order to have perfect health. I guess doctors would be out of a job if we all become more aware of which foods harm us.

Our bodies are a storehouse for the chemical elements. When we experience burn out, the chemical reserves held in our organs are depleted. We then become sick. In order to get back to health, we must pay back what we "owe" the body. This can take a little time, especially if we are a little bit older. This is how I work out how long our recovery process will take: If you are under forty, then take one week for every year you are old, add this up, and this is how long your "back to health" process will take. For example, you are thirty-six years old. So that is thirty-six weeks; divide this by four (to make a month) and you'll get nine. Therefore, it will take nine months of you cleaning out your system, building up your immunity and eating all the right foods and doing some soul-searching for all your reservoirs to be fully nourished again.

Of course, you'll feel better within two weeks of doing this, but keep going. Take a good look at your iris, take a picture, and watch how your colour will change to deeper blue or clearer brown.

For those who have green or hazel eyes your true colour is blue. You were born with blue eyes but shortly after your eyes started changing colour. You inherited this from your family and also the underactive bowel that comes with green and hazel eyes. If you would do this cleanse twice as long then you'll start to see blue underneath which is your true colour.

If you're over forty, it will take two weeks for every year you've been alive to be totally healed. We can simplify this by taking the age and dividing by two instead of four to get the number of weeks. For example, if you are forty-two years old, divide this by two. Therefore, it will take twenty-one months to be totally healed. When you are over forty, it takes so much longer because often we have already become stiff and have signs of arthritis and aging. To fully reverse this process, we must top up our chemical elements 100 percent. Take this time to reconnect with yourself; read books, join groups that will nourish your soul. Do this for yourself. Take your time, and don't be hard on yourself; be patient. You will age without crooked fingers, you'll stay flexible, and you'll stay youthful mentally as well as physically. The best thing you can do for yourself is to study nutrition (not diet).

> Foods build specific systems in our body. Foods contain chemical elements high in the minerals supporting this system. Twelve systems are responsible for carrying on the life process in the human body. These are the skeletal, muscular, respiratory, endocrine, digestive, reproductive, integumentary, lymphatic, excretory, circulatory, nervous and urinary systems. Disease preys on an undernourished person.
>
> —Dr. Bernard Jensen

Often our thinking habits can exhaust our chemical reserves. Sometimes we must change ourselves or even our environment to become healthy again. There are people who go through life not knowing that through their own negative thinking, they are destroying themselves and influencing others around them. This depletes the nervous system. It brings out rashes and lowers the immune system. Not good! Better to change the environment. We must live in peaceful circumstances within ourselves and with those around us. Our human psychology and body chemistry are related. Poor food habits result in nutritional deficiencies in the brain, leading to mental disease, including addiction. Therefore it is important to choose the right foods.

The properties found in foods are either alkaline or acidic. Alkalinity makes strong bases, and when we have a base with a negative, then it is acidic. When these bases engage with our stomach acids, there is a chemical warfare between them. They are opposites. To restore health and to remain in health, we must have alkalinity to neutralize acidity in our stomach.

> *"You may be looking for a good doctor. I am looking for a good patient!"*
>
> *—Dr. Bernard Jensen*

The most alkaline food is sodium; next comes magnesium. Potassium is alkaline to our muscles and urinary system. Calcium is alkaline to the bones. Magnesium is alkaline to the brain, and iron to the blood. Sodium is alkaline to the alimentary tract.

This alkaline principle in foods can cure most diseases without doctors or pills. Please note: Salt is *not* a sodium food. We get sodium from spinach, celery, okra, carrots and strawberries, not sugar or chocolate-dipped strawberries, and not cooked spinach or cooked carrots. If you do cook them, you'll get spinach and carrots minus the sodium.

> *"Chemical elements that are alkaline are most valuable for the sick man, and foods that are acidic are very bad for the sick man."*
>
> *—Dr. Bernard Jensen*

So, why did I become a vegan? Well, over time, my reasons for living this lifestyle changed. It began because I didn't want to eat my animal friends when I was five years old after the kiddie animal farm. Then it changed to the fact that factory farming is simply so wrong on so many levels. Then my focus changed to being environmental and political when I saw a program where rich Europeans were chopping down virgin forests in the Amazon to make clear land to grow food crops, *not* to feed the hungry children but the factory animals back home. Also, the huge amounts of pollution produced by the animal farming industry, in the growing, feeding and killing of animals. To me, it is all so unnecessary, especially as I studied nutrition. I knew we didn't need to eat meat in order to be healthy. In fact, we don't need to eat animal protein for any reason. Every animal protein is acidic, from fish to dairy. Now I've come to a stage in my life where I just want peace of mind. My reasons have become more spiritual, and I have become Vegan.

> *"Truth alone will endure, all the rest will be swept away before the tide of time. Mine may be a voice in the wilderness, but it will be heard when all other voices are silenced. It is the voice of the Truth. Be the change you want to see."*
> —*Mahatma Gandhi*

I stopped eating dairy a long time ago, although I would still eat the occasional biscuit. I want to eat "cruel free" food. That means I also don't eat chocolate or foods containing palm oil. I don't want to bring suffering to this world, whether it is to man or animal. It means I keep my driving to a minimum. I plant trees to offset my carbon usage when I have to fly. I grow as much of my own food as is possible. I do not buy cotton clothes because of the enormous pollution it creates.

On a spiritual level, I understand that life is about suffering, but we can prevent being the cause of suffering. That is why we have to keep on learning. We have to be aware. We need to look at ways that we can become better people. We cannot be oblivious to what is happening to our world, whether you believe in global warming or not. Improve yourself. Work on your own karma.

> *"How people treat you is their karma; how you react is yours."*
> —*Wayne W. Dyer*

There is no justifiable reason to eat meat. Go on, ask yourself why you eat it. Because you like it? Wow, isn't that a little childish? Children want their lollies, sweets and candies, but as adults, we know better. We know it rots their teeth away. We understand they "like" it, but do they need it? No, in fact it is bad for them. As adults, we should think about meat in the same way and know where our meat came from and what it takes for the animal being to be on our plate. We have to acknowledge the cruelty that goes on in our dairy industry.

Are you really all right with being part of all this because you "like" it? "What about our farmers?" I hear you say. "Our farmers are making a living out of this." Well, let me take you back not so long ago when people performed all the manual labour in every factory and industry. There were no computers or machines to do our work for us. When the threat of computers entering the workforce became real, we all panicked. It was a very scary time, because we saw a very real reason for us to lose our jobs. There were many demonstrations worldwide, because millions of people were going to lose their jobs. In any typical factory where hundreds of men worked, they were replaced by a computerized machine that was operated by just one or two men.

You know what happened? It was all right. The change was gradual, and other jobs were created, and the millions who did lose their jobs were integrated somewhere else and in a different way. We saw this on a much smaller scale when our government decided to stop logging some forests in Tasmania. Our loggers lost their jobs, but you know what happened? The remaining forests were turned into National Parks and created lots of tourism. Financially, it brought in far more revenue from tourism than logging, and many of the men who were first making a living out of cutting the forest down are now working in the National Parks, helping to maintain the health of these forests.

Life is change, and change is gradual. The people who work at factory farms, own farms, and make a living out of suffering will find other ways to make money. They will be all right. If millions of men are all right after the introduction of computers, then a few thousand farmers and factory farmers will be all right as well. People don't like change, even if it is for the better. Change is often forced upon us; it is rarely voluntary. Life is change. Go with the flow, and if the flow is towards veganism, then look into it.

> Lean into Veganism. It is much easier this way when you gently "lean" into it.
>
> —Kathy Freston

After the age of forty-five, we should eat less, and we should become more fussy with the foods we eat. This is the time to cut out junk foods. Make your own juice in a cold juicer, also known as slow juicers. They grind the juice out of the fruit and vegetables. The motor stays cold, keeping the minerals intact. I would not use the strainer, as the little bit of pulp in the juice is fibre, which we need very much. Drink your juice straight away. Every second counts, as light and oxygen rob the juice of its vitamins and minerals. Collect the pulp that is left, and feed it to your worms, compost it or make it into patties. They are very nice; give it a go. The best juice you can have is celery, carrots, parsley, beetroot and cucumber. Do not mix fruit and vegetables together.

In the morning, fruit juice is most desirable. Apple, berries and kiwifruit are great. Watermelon should be juiced by itself, and juice the seeds as well. Pineapple, guava and pawpaw are also a good combination. In the afternoon, vegetable juices are more favourable. Do eat at least 60 percent raw, and if you are sick, cut out proteins. If this sickness was caused by diet, then the only way to cure it is by diet. It means you have neglected the foods that keep you well. To fully cure, you must build a new man. We make new cells all the time. New cells build new stomachs, new hearts, new bones, brain and organs.

That is the only way you can be cured, by methods of cell development and purification. Give these cells the right chemical elements, so they can carry out in harmony the rebuilding of a new body. Indeed, if we would live on foods that prevent viruses and contagious diseases by making our immunity strong, then flu shots or vaccinations would be unnecessary.

Doctors are making a living from ignorant people.

> *"The doctor who pays no attention to diet is not a desirable doctor, and you should not request his services."*
>
> *—Dr. Bernard Jensen*

Do you remember what the vegans of the 1960s and '70s looked like? They were anaemic, thin and unhealthy-looking. We called them hippies, and for all their good intensions, they looked tired. Those kind of vegans don't exist anymore. Cells need time to change. Global-consciousness energy levels need to be raised. The Earth's energy levels needed to rise, in order for these courageous souls to function healthier in our Western society. Those in the East who have led a vegan lifestyle for centuries are already there in the higher consciousness. Being a vegan doesn't mean that you just give up meat. It means living a life with a higher consciousness.

Veganism needs to become a lifestyle. Not all human energies can handle this purity and therefore go back to eating animal beings. When we take animal proteins out of our body's system, we make room for inner growth, and that needs time.

One must live the way he preaches. When we are used to eating animal beings and we stop for a little while, our body will start craving meat. Women usually experience these cravings around their menstrual cycle. Why is this? This is because our cells are changing. The animal proteins are leaving the body, and just like other addictions that we give up, the brain will tell the body to fill up again with meat. Think about sugar cravings. They only happen when sugar leaves the body and levels are low. Think about cigarettes. You only have cravings when nicotine is low in the body. We can become violently ill when we give things up. Coffee will give you a headache if you missed out on your usual morning cuppa. So will the absence of meat. Educate yourself; it is going to mean the difference between becoming healthy or staying stuck in an unhealthy lifestyle.

Be kind to yourself; you are on the right path.

> *"Once you come to terms with why you don't eat cats, dogs, monkeys, and dolphins, you'll begin to understand why I don't eat cows, pigs, chickens and lambs."*
>
> *—Edward Sanchez*

For those who are gardeners, what do you do if your soil is too acidic or too alkaline? You feed it! You feed it organic compost, in order to bring the pH back into balance. If our personal pH is too acidic, we need organic greens to bring our system in balance again. We need to feed our bodies the right stuff to grow healthy cells. Cells need to be able to get all the essential nutrition from fruit, vegetables, grains, seeds, nuts, sprouts and legumes.

A meat-eating body is an acidic body, and this is where we see the biggest change… Giving up "dead" food and replacing it with "live" food will make our bodies alkaline. One needs to educate oneself enough to replace meat with a rich, nutritious diet. An acidic body is addicted to acidic food and drinks. An alkaline body rejects acidic food and drinks. So this in itself is a huge change for the person. An alkaline body does not want chips, chocolate, fast food, cola and sweets. Wouldn't that be nice, to get to that stage?

When acidity moves through the body through the process of elimination, we will feel "out of sorts" with ourselves. It is hard to focus on the tasks of the day, we want to sleep, and our speech makes no sense or is slurred. We start hearing crackling noises in our inner ear, neck and sinus areas. But then, our neck starts loosening up. Our joints can hurt. We have sleepless nights and loss of appetite. We can experience all of this when we give up acidic food. We crave sugar, but hopefully with the newfound knowledge of how bad sugar is for us, we can refrain from it.

Those who have done an internal cleanse know this feeling. We cannot concentrate, as we feel like we are in a fog. Hopefully, with the knowledge of how bad acidic foods are for us, we can refrain from eating them while our systems become balanced. Then the brain fog goes, and we feel we see everything more clearly, especially on a spiritual level. Our senses of sight and smell are more sensitive, and we can hear better. All this happens when a person goes through this change. The first time is the worst time. It takes about three days for this process to evolve.

The body then gets used to the change, and a newfound energy replaces the old sluggish feeling, especially around 3:00 p.m. How nice would it be not to be tired at that time of day!

You will start waking up feeling rested, happy, and looking forward to the day. What's more, you can jump up without feeling stiff in your joints and needing time to get up to speed.

> "When diet is wrong, medicine is of no use.
> When diet is correct, medicine is of no need."
> —Ayurvedic proverb

What has this to do with being a vegan? Well, all animal protein is acidic—every animal protein! It doesn't matter if it is fish, dairy, a steak or honey, it all turns our system acidic. "But," I hear you say, "we are allowed 20 percent acidity in our diet every day." Yes, but animal protein is the wrong kind of acidity. What we are talking about is the example of, let's say, a lemon. This is definitely an acidic fruit, but when it hits our stomach and digestive system, it alkalises it. It builds an alkaline cell in our stomach wall.

When we talk about 20 percent acidity, we mean cranberries, corn, walnuts and tomatoes. Our 10 percent acidic protein and 10 percent starch that we recommend is brown rice, barley, lentils, nuts, and a range of beans and tahini. For starch products, we recommend, potatoes, brown rice, bananas, sweet potatoes, yams, corn, legumes, pumpkin, organic pita bread and couscous. With potatoes, I recommend not having them too often. In fact, the less you have, the better. It is a nightshade vegetable. (I write about nightshade vegetables later.)

If you must have potatoes, try to keep the skins on; don't boil them, and eat them cold, as in a potato salad. Eat sweet potatoes, yams and pumpkin instead. The difference is that these foods are acidic, but in our system it alkalises our stomach walls. Animal protein is acidic, but it acidifies our stomach. It actually strips the alkalinity from our system. It takes a lot of greens to balance that out again. This also goes for all junk food, sugar, and alcohol, coffee, tea, supermarket juices and soft drinks. All these foods are acidic and strip our body of alkalinity from the stomach walls. Junk food is not food at all; it is just junk!

People on vegan diets have high-alkaline diets, which promotes health and youthfulness.

> *"Children are scared of the dark, and adults are scared of the light."*
>
> *—adapted from Plato*

The research into veganism continues. I guess this is a good thing, but to me, it is common sense to eat what is right for you. We know that fried food, donuts, coffee, soda and junk food are extremely bad for us. We don't need research to tell us that, but we continue to consume these products, giving power to these companies that supply our needs more and more each year. What really rubs me the wrong way is when, from time to time, when researchers feel compelled to prove a point that is far from the truth. Soymilk and soy products are a classic example. Every time an article comes out to prove how bad soy is, people who never studied nutrition or soy products say, "See how bad it is?" Yes, it is bad for the meat and dairy industry! It is never an independent researcher who wrote this article, but usually government departments, meat or diary industries or medical companies sponsored by pharmaceuticals. None of these people has your best interest in mind because it will affect their wealth. There is an excellent article written by doctor Holly Wilson MD called soy Myths and Misinformation. Please Google this and read it. The other thing is that some people who make snap judgements about soy products happily drink coffee and Coke and happily eat donuts and fried foods.

Let me ask you something: Close your eyes and imagine a typical Aussie man. What does he look like? Does he look like a person who would drink soymilk and eat tofu? No, I didn't think so.

Now close your eyes again. Imagine a typical man who drinks soymilk and eats tofu. Does this man look fitter, skinnier and healthier?

The truth is that people who consume soy products do not drink litres of soymilk. They use a little in their tea (rooibos, of course). They eat a little organic tofu now and again. They eat tempeh and maybe veggie burgers or veggie sausages at a barbeque. These products are readily available in organic varieties and don't cost much. People who consume soymilk certainly do not get the mucus that cow's milk produces; it doesn't give us earaches or snotty noses. Please always buy organic tofu or tempeh and soymilk, and please educate yourself on the benefits and also how to cook with it, even if you are a flesh-eater.

> *"Have a mouth as sharp as a dagger, but a heart as soft as tofu."*
> *—Chinese proverb*

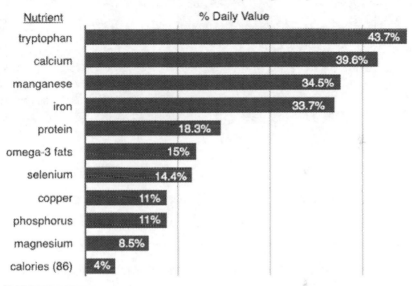

Nutrients in Tofu (113 grams)

Nutrient	% Daily Value
tryptophan	43.7%
calcium	39.6%
manganese	34.5%
iron	33.7%
protein	18.3%
omega-3 fats	15%
selenium	14.4%
copper	11%
phosphorus	11%
magnesium	8.5%
calories (86)	4%

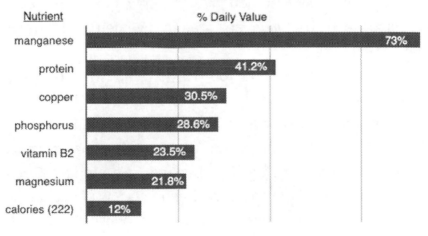

Nutrients in Tempeh (113 grams)

Nutrient	% Daily Value
manganese	73%
protein	41.2%
copper	30.5%
phosphorus	28.6%
vitamin B2	23.5%
magnesium	21.8%
calories (222)	12%

"I've been vegan for fifteen years, and it turns out it makes a very big impact on the environment to eat fewer animal products, which cause more greenhouse gases than all of transportation combined. The United Nations did a study just over two years ago, and that blew my mind. I started thinking that if people are vegetarian for just one day a week, that makes a huge difference!"

—Emily Deschanel

My own story

When you are almost fifty years of age, doctors feel compelled to examine you, to see how healthy you are and make you aware of all the bad things that will start to happen to you in the near future. So, I first went in to see a male doctor, who frowned upon the fact that I am vegan. He asked if I drank soymilk, and I said yes. He then proceeded to tell me how bad soy was for me. My first thought was, *Wow, here is a doctor who knows about nutrition,* so I was mildly interested to hear what he had to say.

Then there was a knock on his door, and his secretary walked in and gave him a big mug of black coffee. He had lost my interest right there and then. If he was happy to drink coffee, then he was not the right person to tell me how bad soymilk was. He said that soy should be banned as a product. Does he also think Coca-Cola should be banned? How about Maccy D's? Refined and processed foods? Sugar, white flour, white rice, meat, fish, dairy products, donuts, fried foods, salt, chips, alcohol, yeast, pasta, coffee, black tea, chocolate, sweets, fatty foods, white bread, pastries, canned foods, sweetened juices, additives and preservatives? Does he think that all this also should be banned? Personally, I would give up all these products before I would give up tofu and soymilk.

The problem he had with soy is that soy contains trypsin Inhibitors. Trypsin is produced in the pancreas and enables the uptake of protein in our food. Trypsin predigests protein. However, trypsin inhibitors are only present in *raw* soy protein. As soon as it is cooked, it deactivates the block and becomes an easily digestible food.

Besides that, there are heaps of foods that are trypsin-prohibitory, including any food that has egg white in it. Also lima beans and breast milk. The other so-called problem the doctor had with soy is that it contains goitrogens. Goitrogens interfere with the thyroid gland by suppressing the iodine uptake. Virtually every plant we eat has compounds that contain goitrogens, but these same plants have many other compounds that counteract goitrogens. Seaweed is a good example, as it does contain a very weak goitrogenic effect, but also contains a strong iodine effect, which counteracts the goitrogens.

Goitrogens are also found in broccoli, kale, cabbage and cauliflower, caffeine, strawberries, pine nuts, pears, bamboo shoots, bokchoy and many other foods... The doctor picked soy to tell me about interference with thyroid function. Fermented food also has goitrogens.

Yes, there is a sick-thyroid epidemic happening in Western cultures, but it is not due to tofu! Deleting foods that suppress the thyroid is crazy, not to mention it is still lacking iodine. Continual stress, sadness, depression, sugar, coffee, pollution, alcohol and exhaustion all cause the thyroid to malfunction. I encourage people to eat foods high in iodine, like dulse (purple seaweed), kombu, nori, okra, and celery.

> *"It is no measure of health to be well adjusted to a profoundly sick society."*
>
> *-Jiddu Krishnamurti*

Needless to say, I did not have this doctor check me out. Instead, I went to a female doctor who gave me all the possible tests. She knew quiet a lot about nutrition and was very interested in the fact that I was a vegan. She asked if there were any books she could read on the subject. I returned two weeks later for the results, and I came out shining! I was not low in anything. She told me that I was very fit and my health was above average for my age.

So, in future, when you read about soymilk and its dangers, always find out who wrote it, and you'll see it is for their own benefit, whoever it may be. I must say, if you do drink soymilk or eat tofu, always make sure that it is organic. There is rice milk, oat milk, hemp and almond milk as well, so drink a variety of them.

> *"A 2012 analysis of all the best studies done to date concluded vegetarians have significantly lower cancer rates. For example, the largest forward-looking study on diet and cancer ever performed concluded that "the incidence of all cancers combined is lower among vegetarians."*
>
> *—Kathy Freston*

Health benefits of tofu are varied. It is rich in vegetable protein, it contains all eight essential amino acids, it's low in saturated fats and carbohydrates, and it is cholesterol free. It is an excellent source of calcium, fibre, linoleic acid (which helps to clear the arteries), lecithin, vitamins B and E, choline, iron, potassium and phosphorus. In Southeast Asia, where tofu is an important part of the daily diet, people are less prone to heart disease; cancers of the prostate, breast and ovaries; osteoporosis and menopausal symptoms.

In addition to this, tofu is free of high levels of chemical toxins which are found in meat, dairy and fish proteins. Dairy and meat products are the most concentrated source of toxins, since they are high in fat and most of the poisons that find their way into the food chain are fat-soluble. This depletes calcium, overworks the liver and kidneys, stagnates digestion and destroys our good bacteria. It leads to kidney stones, colon and bowel disorders, constipation, arthritis, osteoporosis and heart disease. It triggers allergic responses such as sinusitis, asthma, earache, congestion, runny nose, skin rashes, eczema, fatigue, lethargy and irritability.

Animal protein acidifies the blood and puts a strain on the body's ability to produce enzymes and hydrochloric acid, which are necessary for digestion.

So give me tofu anytime. At least it is digestible. Have it with your greens in stir-fries, in soups, in salads or just by itself, accompanied by your veggies.

> *"Tell me what you eat, and I will tell you who you are."*
> —*Brillat-Savarin*

Comparisons

Still think we are meant to eat meat?

Here are some comparisons between meat-eating animals, herbivores and humans.

Meat-eaters: have claws
Herbivores:　 no claws
Humans:　　 no claws

Meat-eaters: have no skin pores and perspire through the tongue
Herbivores:　 perspire through skin pores
Humans:　　 perspire through skin pores

Meat-eaters: have sharp front teeth for tearing, and no flat molar teeth for grinding.
Herbivores:　 no sharp front teeth, but flat rear molars for grinding.
Humans:　　 no sharp front teeth, but flat rear molars for grinding.

Meat-eaters: have intestinal tract that is only three times their body length so that rapidly decaying meat can pass through quickly.
Herbivores:　 have intestinal tract ten to twelve times their body length.
Humans:　　 have intestinal tract ten to twelve times their body length.

Meat-eaters: have strong hydrochloric acid in stomach to digest meat.

Herbivores: have stomach acid that is twenty times weaker than that of a meat-eater.

Humans: have stomach acid that is twenty times weaker than that of a meat-eater.

The bowels of humans and carnivores are strikingly different.

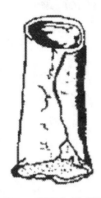

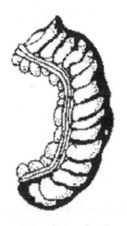

Portion of a typical carnivore bowel   Portion of a typical human bowel

> "If you have men who will exclude any of God's creatures from the shelter of compassion and pity, you will have men who will deal likewise with their fellow men."
> —St. Francis of Assisi

Meat-eaters: salivary glands in mouth not needed to predigest grains and fruits.

Herbivores: well-developed salivary glands which are necessary to predigest grains and fruits.

Humans: well-developed salivary glands, which are
             necessary to predigest grains and fruits.

Meat-eaters: have acid saliva with no enzyme ptyalin to predigest
             grains.
Herbivores: have alkaline saliva with ptyalin to predigest grains.
Humans: have alkaline saliva with ptyalin to predigest grains.

Based on a chart by A.D. Andrews, Fit Food for Men, (Chicago:
American Hygiene Society, 1970)

In addition, there are other comparisons: meat-eaters like lions sleep most of the day, in order to have the energy to sprint to kill their prey. Vegetarian animals (us included) are awake all day. We tend to graze, eat when we are hungry, and our energy is spread across the day. We need to have our reserves up in order to have energy to do anything where as meateaters hunt when they are hungry. Meateaters also are happy to eat every two or three days. We are just too different from anything on Earth that eats meat. Meat-eaters must have their food raw. When a deer is burned in a forest fire, wolves do not eat it, and when lions are fed cooked meat, they become sick.

The lifespan of all vegetarians is much longer in the animal world, as well as with us.

Mammal	Years
Elephant	69
Hippopotamus	49
Chimpanzee	40
Grizzly Bear	32

Horse	32
Bison	30
Elk	22
Cow	20
Beaver	19
Wolf	16
Squirrel	16

Lions in the wild live to about ten to sixteen years. In zoos, they can live up to twenty-five years. Dogs and cats live up to fifteen years. The giant tortoise lives to 152 years and the box turtle lives to 123 years old.

These animals eat mostly grasses, leaves, fruits, flowers, seeds, herbs and woody stems.[2]

My point is that pure meat-eaters don't live as long, compared to all other animals, including us.

While we're comparing physical differences, let's consider teeth in more depth. People love to say, "I wouldn't have canines if I weren't meant to eat meat." I say, "Have you ever seen the canines of a gorilla?" They're much bigger and stronger than ours, and they're used primarily for eating fruits, vegetables, seeds, and nuts. Gorillas sometimes eat ants, but they never use their canines to eat meat. Besides that, humans and gorillas only have four incisors, whereas dogs, cats, lions, and polar bears have twelve incisors.

Our ancestors used tools like spears to kill animals. We had to use our brain rather than rely on our speed, strength, claws and teeth to kill.

"Man's structure, external and internal, compared with that of other animals, show that fruit and succulent vegetables constitute his natural food." Much of the world still lives that way. Even in most industrialized countries, the love affair with meat is less than a hundred years old. It started with the refrigerator and car and the twentieth-century consumer society. But even with the twentieth century, man's body hasn't adapted to eating meat

—Swedish scientist Karl von Linne

Humans are Herbivores

	Carnivores	Omnivores	Herbivores	Humans
Teeth: Incisors	Short and pointed	Short and pointed	Flat and wide	Flat and wide
Teeth: Canines	round, long and sharp	round, long and sharp	None, short or long for defense and blunt	short and blunt
Teeth: Molars	Sharp, jagged and blade-shaped	Sharp blades and or flat teeth	Flat with cusps	Flat with nodular cusps.
Major Jaw Muscles	Large	Large	Small	Small
Chewing	none, as food is swallowed whole	none, as food is swallowed whole	Must chew food before swallowing	Must chew food before swallowing
Digestive system - Colon	Short straight and smooth	Short straight and smooth	Long and complex with segmented appearance	Long with segmented appearance
pH of foods	suits acidic foods	can have acidic foods	only eat alkaline foods and a very small amount of acidic foods.	only suit alkaline foods with a very small amount of acidic foods.
pH of stomach acidity	pH 1 - 2	pH 1 - 2	pH 4-5	pH 4-5
Health problems	No health problems by eating meat	No health problems by eating meat	Animal protein leads to a weak constitution	Animal protein leads to a weak constitution
Nails	Sharp claws	Sharp claws	Flat nails or hooves	Flat nails
Kidney	Urine is extremely concentrated	Urine is extremely concentrated	Urine is moderately concentrated	Urine is moderately concentrated
Jaw joint location	On the same plane as molar teeth	On the same plane as molar teeth	Above the plane of molars	Above the plane of molars
Jaw motion	up and down	up and down	side to side	side to side

Carnivore	Herbivore	Human
has claws	no claws	no claws
no pores on skin; perspires through tongue to cool body	perspires through millions of pores on skin	perspires through millions of pores on skin
sharp, pointed front teeth to tear flesh	no sharp, pointed front teeth	no sharp, pointed front teeth
no flat back molar teeth to grind food	has flat, back molar teeth to grind food	has flat, back molar teeth to grind food
small salivary glands in the mouth (not needed to pre-digest grains and fruits)	well-developed salivary glands needed to pre-digest grains and fruits	well-developed salivary glands needed to pre-digest grains and fruits
acid saliva	alkaline saliva	alkaline saliva
strong hydrochloric acid in stomach to digest tough animal muscle, bone, etc.	stomach acid 20 times weaker than that of meat-eaters	stomach acid 20 times weaker than that of meat-eaters
intestinal tract only 3 times body length, so rapidly decaying meat can pass out of body quickly	intestinal tract several times body length, so body can absorb maximum nutrients from plant food decay	intestinal tract several times body length, so body can absorb maximum nutrients from plant food decay

What Is Making You Unwell?

Certain thoughts have certain effects on the body. Many diseases started in the mind, and many diseases healed when a person's thinking was changed. Louise Hay wrote *You Can Heal Your Life*. If you have it, then it is a good book to read again, and if you don't have it, the library will.

Fear, hate and anger can cause congestion, resulting in an excessive amount of blood gathering in some parts of the body. Therefore, a clot or even a stroke can happen. That is why fear, stress and anger can give you high blood pressure. Anger and anxiety affect the adrenal glands, and great sadness affects the thyroid glands, which is the emotional gland. The thyroid and the liver are connected. A person with thyroid problems also has liver problems. Therefore, you can understand that good thinking is good for the liver.

The body is always the effect, never the cause! Many people need a new way of thinking and new foods to go with it. Old food patterns keep people stagnant.

> *"It is not happy people who are thankful, It is thankful people who are happy."*
>
> *—author unknown*

Change your foods, and you will change your way of thinking. Humans must grow; we must change; we must embrace new challenges and thought patterns, and new foods will allow this process to happen. When we fall back on old eating habits, it is our old way of thinking that puts us there. Often, our old foods don't taste the same way anymore, and it is a disappointment.

Why? Because we have grown out of old patterns for a while, and this has changed our taste buds. Taking care of our mind is harder than taking care of our body.

Look back ten years, even five or two years. Can you honestly say that you have not grown? I bet that some old beliefs are gone or have evolved. I bet some opinions have changed. I bet that your diet has changed as well. How many people say, "I don't eat (something like fatty chips) like I used to." Why is that? Because mentally and spiritually, we have grown. We extended our vision for ourselves. We don't *make* this happen on purpose, but we *let* this happen. We don't force anything; we let change happen. It is when we are stubborn, headstrong and angry that the flow stops. We need to have trust and let the flow of life happen.

> *"The body is always the effect, never the cause."*
> —*Dr. Bernard Jensen*

Through iridology, we've been able to compare many people's behaviours, lifestyles and thinking patterns and draw conclusions between the health of their minds and the health of their physical bodies. You must look at the whole person. Thoughts and feelings are very important. You cannot just treat the physical body. As an example, we had a lady come to the clinic who wanted an iridology reading. She was slim and fit, and her diet was close to perfect. She ate the correct food combinations, ratios of 80 percent alkaline and 20 percent acidic, ate 60 percent raw, and most of it was organic. On paper, you couldn't get a better, healthier lifestyle. Yet she didn't feel right; she felt heavy with no energy.

When we took a look in her eyes, we noticed that her head area was extremely acidic. It told us that she was thinking way too much, and she was thinking a lot of negative thoughts. She was not grateful for much in her life. She was stressed at work, and her relationship was testing. Her stomach was acidic and foggy. She did not have the deep-blue eyes, which comes with an alkaline diet like hers. Her eyes told us that she was in pain, and she was. She was miserable. Miserable in her marriage, in her workplace, but most of all, she was miserable within herself. She was angry and disappointed in life. No amount of carrot juice is going to fix that. So how *do* you fix that?

She had been taking care of the outer person very well— the outer physical body. She never addressed the inner person. We are talking about her inner happiness, her feelings, beliefs and peace of mind. Where was she at with her spiritual search? Unhappiness will be found in the physical process in the body. She needed to learn to meditate, write things down, forgive, communicate and most of all be truthful. What she needed to become a healthy person, she could not get from me. She needed soul-searching for that. She needed to clean up her mind first, because the body will be a servant to wherever the mind is.

If you want to get out of your physical troubles, you will have to raise your mind to a higher level of thinking.

> *"'Don't beat yourself up over things.' WELL, DO!!!*
> *Find out exactly where those feelings come from, dig deep.*
> *Not to beat ourselves up is not to self examine ourselves."*
> *—Dierk Kimler*

My Favourite Story: There was once a time when all human beings were gods, but they so abused their divinity that Brahma, the chief god, decided to take it away from them and hide it where it could never be found. Where to hide their divinity was the question. So Brahma called a council of the gods to help them decide. "Let's bury it deep in the earth," said the gods, but Brahma answered, "No, that will not do, because humans will dig into the earth and find it."

Then the gods said, "Let's sink it in the deepest ocean." But Brahma said, "No, not there, for they will learn to dive into the ocean and will find it."

Then the gods said, "let's take it to the top of the highest mountain and hide it there." But once again Brahma replied, "No, that will not do either, because they will eventually climb every mountain and once again take up their divinity."

Then the gods gave up and said, "We do not know where to hide it, because it seems that there is no place on earth or in the sea that human beings will not eventually reach."

Brahma thought for a long time and then said, "Here is what we will do. We will hide their divinity deep in the centre of their own being, for humans will never think to look for it there." All the gods agreed that this was the perfect hiding place, and the deed was done. And since that time, humans have been going up and down the earth, digging, diving, climbing and exploring—searching for something already within themselves.

We need to be calm, and we need to go within. We need to meditate in order to "know thyself." This takes practice. Therefore, for your own good, you need to love. Health is made up of many good thoughts.

If we are going to have peace within our bodies, then we will first have to have peace within our minds. Why is this? Because the mind is the bridge between the spiritual and the physical. We must learn never to quarrel or to argue. We must learn to communicate honestly. Do not associate with negative people. Pick your companions with care, and bring out the best in them. This all takes work. We are all free to make our own choices and search for truths. Through searching, right thinking and right living, we can redirect our lives to the highest level possible. Our beliefs determine our reality to a very great extent; therefore, people can change their lives just by changing the direction of their thinking. If you can change your life mentally, you can easily change your life physically.

> "Wisdom comes at the end of our experiences."
>
> —Sacha Guitry

Stress and Proper Digestion

Have you ever thought about why you cannot eat when you have a knot in your stomach due to stress? Why you lose your appetite when you've just had an argument with your partner? The brain responds to this stress, and digestion is the last thing it is worried about. Digestion shuts down, together with the glands and organs involved. The body diverts its energy to the respiratory and circulatory systems.

The brain must be alert, to spring into action. This includes emotional stress, stress from injury, surgery and too many toxins.

No harm is done to our physical body if stress happens every now and then. As soon as we've calmed down, digestion starts up again. However, if we are under stress for long periods, the long-term effect is detrimental to our digestive system, resulting in irritable bowel syndrome. People with IBS are unable to digest and absorb the nutrients in their food properly. This condition gives a person a lot of pain in the abdominal area and intestinal wall, with a lot of gas production. The person becomes weaker as their immunity doesn't function properly.

> *"Let food be thy medicine and medicine be thy food."*
> *—Hippocrates*

As of 2012, as many as one in seven people in Australia had been diagnosed with irritable bowel syndrome (IBS). It is suspected that this number would double if all victims were diagnosed. This is what I say to people who claim they have irritable bowel syndrome: "Stop irritating it!" If you have this condition, think about it—stop irritating your bowels with the food and drinks that irritate it in the first place. Change your food choices, drink more water, and be kind to yourself.

You can cure yourself, lose weight and eliminate all foods that caused it in the first place. You must keep to nature's law. If you think you've got a choice or can sneak in a greasy hamburger here and there, well, you *cannot!* You do not have a choice. On page 72 I've written a formula for how long it takes to clean out your system and recover from any illness you've ever had. Here it is again: If you are under forty, take one week for every year you are old; add this up, and this is how long your "back to health" process will take. For example, you are thirty-six years old. So that is thirty-six weeks; divide this by four (to make a month) and you'll get nine.

> *"I don't know a better preparation for life than a love of poetry and a good digestion."*
>
> —*Zona Gale*

Therefore, it will take nine months of you cleaning out your system, building up your immunity, and eating all the right foods and doing some soul-searching for all your reservoirs to be fully nourished again.

If you're over forty, it will take two weeks to heal for every year you've been alive. We can simplify this by taking the age and dividing by two instead of four to get the number of weeks For example, If you are forty-two years old, divide this by two. Therefore, it will take twenty-one months to be totally healed. When you are over forty, it takes so much longer because often we have already become stiff and have signs of arthritis and ageing.

If you are a person who can only go to the toilet after a cup of coffee, think about it—the coffee irritates your bowels. Your body wants to get rid of it as quickly as possible, because coffee causes rectal cancer. It is a no-brainer. Eat lots of fruit instead; it strengthens the bowels.

You cannot be healthy with a sick bowel. A healthy bowel absorbs all nutrients from the foods we eat. In order for this process to occur, we need strong, healthy stomach acid. This is called hydrochloric acid, and its job is to break down foods so that your body can absorb all nutrients. When this acid is deficient through eating the wrong foods, then we become bloated, we burp and we have gas. This all happens when our acids are too weak and the food is not fully digested. It then ferments and produces gas. Yes, better out than in, but if your hydrochloric acid is strong enough, then no gas should be produced. So IBS starts because our acid is too weak, not because it is too strong. Drug companies that say you need to buy acid-suppressing drugs are conning you. You do not have to suppress your acid; you need to feed it, not neutralize it! It is a US $7 billion-per-year industry and growing every year.

When our hydrochloric acid is low we are malnourished. Indigestion is a lack of strong, healthy acid. It should be pH 4 when we rest and pH 3 when we eat. IBS is always due to the food and drinks we've consumed; however, I must say that with an acidic mind, there will always be an acidic body and low hydrochloric acid. A healthy bowel has billions of highly active "good bacteria," and this creates an environment where "bad bacteria" can't prosper. All sick people have bowel disorders; death begins in the bowel.

> *"IBS, Crohn's disease, constipation, diverticulitis, low energy diabetes, boils, candida, and parasites are all ills due to the bowel not performing good enough."*
>
> *—Ron Gellatley*

How to have a healthy bowel

The average person has up to three kilos of unwanted toxic waste stuck to their bowel wall, which sits there fostering unhealthy conditions. Is it any wonder that bowel disease and bowel cancer are on the rise? This "coating" stops the absorption of all nutrients, minerals and vitamins. The coating was at first produced as a protection layer. Let's pretend our bowels are clean. Coffee, dairy products, junk food, pepper and sugars are extremely painful to digest. We would crumple over until we expel the matter down the toilet. But what happens is that when we are children, these foods are introduced to us in small amounts. Slowly, our bowel will grow a protective layer on the inside wall, which allows us to consume these foods and drinks without physically hurting us. If we have small amounts of this, then the layer is thin enough to still allow the absorption of nutrients.

If we eat junk food—too much and too often—this layer becomes so thick, to protect the bowel wall, that nutrients can no longer be absorbed. People who are overweight also suffer from malnutrition. Children who are overweight already have this yucky coating. If your child is in this position, you are killing him due to the lack of vitamins and minerals he receives.

So, what to do? Simple! Introduce apples, carrots, watermelon, grapes and plain water into the diet. The body will not absorb the nutrients at first, but slowly and surely the toxic matter stuck to the bowel wall will loosen. Eat homemade soups; eat light, digestible foods. No more pasta! What do we make children's glue out of? Flour and water. How do we make pasta? Flour and water and salt. You are eating glue every time you put pasta into your mouth. Did you know that the reason two-minute noodles don't stick together is because they coat the noodles with wax? It takes four days for your body to digest and eliminate that wax. It is not a food; it is glue!

Change the balance. Have light, digestible foods five to six days per week, and have whatever you feel like on the other day(s). You get the idea. You'll eat better, lose weight, lose the three-kilo protective layer, and you will once again absorb the nutrition that you need to live a long and happy life. For people who are overweight, even slightly, the culprit is always acidic foods.

> *"The internal absorbing surface area of the bowel is equivalent to half the size of a tennis court."*
>
> —*R. Bowen*

Now, what about people who are not overweight? You can be the right weight but still not be in optimal health. To stay in optimal health, we need to eat alkaline foods. Healthy hydrochloric acid needs alkaline foods in order to digest our foods properly. A balance of three chemical elements is needed more than any other to keep our hydrochloric acid healthy. They are sodium, potassium and calcium. Alkaline sodium foods include celery, okra, watercress, spinach, apples, asparagus, kale, kelp and strawberries. Remember, salt is not a sodium food; it is not even a food. It is very acidic. Acidic sodium is very bad for our bowels. This includes deli meats, gravies, yeast, sun-dried tomatoes, cheeses, snack foods, popcorn, pickled foods, pizzas, breads, noodle soups, chips, sauces and salad dressings. When you make a salad, do not put salad dressing on, and do not put sun-dried tomatoes or olives in it. It ruins the salad's nutritional value.

Alkaline potassium foods include: apples, bananas, apricots, avocados, squash, dark leafy greens, parsley, beetroot and potato peelings.

Alkaline calcium foods include: avocados, broccoli, cauliflower, dulse, kelp, spinach, dried herbs, tahini, tofu and dark leafy greens. Exercise is essential for calcium increase.

Do not get alkaline calcium confused with acidic calcium, like all dairy products, meats and breads. All animal products are acidic, even honey.

So, this is how it works: if there is an alkaline sodium shortage in the bowel, the stomach wall becomes acidic. In order to keep the bowel alkaline as long as possible, the body takes sodium out of the outer joints of our bodies. Sodium keeps calcium soluble; therefore, when sodium is taken out of the joints (let's say the fingers), your fingers will get stiff, because there is no sodium left in the joints. So, people with stiff fingers, arthritis or rheumatism all lack alkaline sodium in the bowel. Without sodium in the joints, the calcium gets hard, and the fingers become stiff. Simple, isn't it? All we need to do is reverse the process. Eat plenty of alkaline sodium foods; the stomach wall will become alkaline again and stop taking the sodium out of the joints, and therefore our fingers will become flexible again.

> *"Arthritis is a nutritional deficiency disease. If we all eat the nutrients we need, we can live out our lives without the misery of arthritis."*
>
> *—Dr. Ruth Yale Long*

Better Out than In

Did you know that your body would not produce gas if the hydrochloric acid in your bowel was healthy? Actually, it is not your body that produces gas; it is the bacteria from the undigested food you ate. If your body has the inability to digest fully, the food ferments, and this is what produces gas. Ever wondered why some people get gas after eating beans, meat, fruit salad, cabbage, or drinking soymilk, and others don't get gas? It is because of how healthy the person is. The healthier the person, the least amount of wind they have. The person who passes wind needs to eat way more greens, to help his body to digest the more difficult-to-digest foods. So, if alkaline sodium is deficient, gas is generated in the intestinal tract. Food decomposition in the stomach results in gas generation.

If bowels are struggling, acidic foods like meat, beans, white rice, bread, flour, biscuits, coffee, tea, chocolate, eggs, processed and refined foods, pies, pastries, canned foods, ice cream, sugar, fried food, tomato sauce or ketchup, boiled vegetables, preservatives and sauces always produce gas. Sodium will stimulate activity of the stomach walls, enhancing digestion.

> *"Passing wind is full of people whispers."*
>
> *—author unknown*

Emotional Ties with Your Food

You have to let go of the foods which make you sick. If you have asthma, diabetes, obesity or arthritis, you must let go mentally of the foods that caused these problems in the first place. This is difficult, because all these foods are addictive. Acidic foods are extremely addictive. You first have to admit that you are addicted. If you are planning to eat the foods that keep you sick, then I cannot help you. I will tell you to cut out dairy, and then you go home and have it anyway. That is a waste of my time, if you ask me. Why come and ask me in the first place if I can make you feel better?

The change must be within you first. Be ready for this change first before you seek help. The good news is that if you are ready and go home and give up dairy completely, then your addiction and ailments will go completely.

> *"Eating crappy food isn't a reward—it's a punishment."*
> *—Drew Carey*

You'll find, though, that you most likely do not like dairy anymore when you do have it, because your body is no longer addicted and will repulse against it. Your taste buds will have changed. Too quickly, people want to hear what will make them healthy but don't recognise the message because they are not mentally ready yet.

These people haven't grown enough. Find out why you are addicted to certain foods. Are you an emotional eater? What can you not let go of? What are you holding on to? Were your habits formed as a child? Can you really still justify that as a reason for your eating habits? Will you be able to replace it with something a bit healthier for you? Find out, and write down your feelings with the view of growing and giving up your foods that you are addicted to. My mentor, Dr. Bernard Jensen, used to say, "You are looking for a good doctor, well I am looking for a good patient." He meant that he would tell his patients how to get better and they did not listen to him.

> "When we give up dieting, we take back something we were often too young to know we had given away: our own voice. Our ability to make decisions about what to eat and when. Our belief in ourselves. Our right to decide what goes into our mouths. Unlike the diets that appear monthly in magazines or the thermal pants that sweat off pounds, unlike a lover or a friend or a car, your body is reliable. It doesn't go away, get lost, stolen. If you will listen, it will speak."
>
> —Geneen Roth

Our brains are made up of ten billion nerve cells that are constantly evaluating and adjusting to what is going on outside and inside ourselves. If we experience something pleasant, every cell of our body knows what is going on. Physically and emotionally, our cells and our well-being will respond to that experience. Every cell in the body responds to the peace and harmony we have in our minds. The same could be said for your cells being aware of being in a position that is unpleasant; a person who works in an abattoir, for example. Don't you think that his well-being is dragged down? The cells in his brain would be very much aware that he is killing an animal being in horrific circumstances. How do you think his nervous system is? God may forgive you of your sins, but your nervous system never will.

If you choose the higher path, you cannot be dragged down by unpleasantness. This person must stop work at the abattoir for his own mental and spiritual well-being. If you are spiritually aware, then you know you cannot bring suffering to those around you, directly or indirectly. You cannot be responsible for dragging another person down through your actions.

"How wonderful it is that nobody needs to wait a single moment before starting to improve the world—by starting to improve their world."

—Anne Frank

If you eat cruel food, then there is always a person who needs to supply it for you. How would you like to have to kill every day, just so someone else could buy the product in the supermarket, while there is so much other food available for them to eat? Do you really think you deserve happy nerve cells when you're the cause of someone else's depleted nervous system? If you are an animal eater, I would really like for you to answer that question for yourself. You do not deserve more in return than what you give out. Where and how are you going to find foods that will give you spiritual peace? You won't find it in packaged foods, donuts or fast foods. You find it in alive foods and in cruel-free foods. Please become aware of your inner well-being. Work on it. Eliminate situations that are stressful, and be aware of how that makes you feel. Now extend this to your environment.

"There are the waves and there is the wind, seen and unseen forces. Everyone has these same elements in their lives, the seen and unseen, karma and free will."

—Kuan Yin

Be aware of how your actions affect others. Do your actions cause others stress, directly or indirectly? Think about it. As you become more enlightened, can you really continue to cause unhappiness, directly or indirectly?

Small actions have huge effects. An example of this is palm oil. Palm oil is used in thousands of products. We now know that the use of palm oil is the direct cause of deforestation, which is the direct cause of orangutans losing their home and fight for survival. So much devastation, just because we buy products with palm oil in them. Our small act of "goodness" could be that instead of buying peanut butter with palm oil in it, we change to another brand that does not have palm oil in it. If 7 billion people don't buy products with palm oil in them, the forests will stay, and the orangutan will survive. Please look on the Internet to learn more about this subject.

Little positive changes will benefit your nervous system. You will positively influence those around you. They, in return, will feel good about their actions also. It is all about raising the bar and helping those around us raise the bar also. Not everyone is going to be interested. You are going to be responsible for turning to all that is good in life. The more you look to "good," the more you'll find ways to do good. This is one way to work on our spiritual enlightenment.

Our purpose in life is to serve. Find ways to serve, even if it is as small and simple as changing to peanut butter without palm oil in it. We must practice accepting change. With that comes the practice of eating cruel-free foods but also stress-free foods.

Spices are among the harshest things for the nervous system. Pepper is seventeen times more irritating to the liver than alcohol. Spices destroy the nerve endings in the body. Salt, nutmeg, ginger, garlic and other condiments have no food value whatsoever. There is a difference between using these spices for cooking and using them in the proper way as a medicinal plant. For example: garlic should be used in case of worms or a cold. You can lightly steam garlic in order to clean out your system. This is very different from using garlic in your cooking. When it gets too hot, it will lose all its medicinal value and become putrid in the body.

"A nickel will get you on the subway, but garlic will get you a seat."

—Yiddish proverb

Ginger is the same; use it fresh for its medicinal properties, but to fry it on high heat destroys all good, and it becomes irritable to the stomach. Have it raw in soups and stews but add it at the end and don't heat it up too much.

Chocolate is another one that the brain tricks you into thinking it's good to have. Chocolate producers have taken advantage of the fact that it has antioxidants and it improves consumers' mood. Chocolate is addictive, and if you have it, then you really should ask yourself why. It has a lot of sugar. If you are overweight, do not have chocolate anymore. It has a lot of caffeine; do you really choose to give this to your kids? It causes calcium loss, because the high sugar (or any level of sugar, for that matter) will leach calcium out of the body. It is very acidic. The elevation in blood sugar from chocolate also triggers migraines. Chocolate contains oxalates, which give you kidney stones. It gives you acne. People who crave chocolate have magnesium deficiency. Eat plenty of nuts and brown rice (soaking method) okra, corn, leafy green vegetables, seeds and whole grains, and your cravings will diminish. Let your last piece of chocolate be your last piece of chocolate, and never ever give it to your kids.

"Move out of your comfort zone. You can only grow if you are willing to feel awkward and uncomfortable when you try something new."

—Overcoming Addiction
quote by Brian Tracy (born 1944)

Foodless Food

When is food not a food? Well, junk food is the obvious one. Junk food is just junk. Other foods are not so simple to categorize in this way, because we tend to eat lots of them every day, and we are still alive. There are a couple of indicators of nonfood: Does it go off? If the food you are about to eat does *not* go off, then don't eat it. Food that has come from nature will go off if you don't eat it in time. This is the food you want; the fresher the better. Secondly, does your food come in a packet with numbers on it? Do not eat food that has numbers on its packaging. Natural flavours include blood, seafood, meat, fermentation products, MSG, bugs and animal fat. If you think I am joking, take a look at the "natural flavours" that were found in an everyday strawberry milkshake: amyl acetate, amyl butyrate, amyl valerate, anethol, anisyl formate, benzyl acetate, benzyl isobutyrate, butyric acid, cinnamyl isobutyrate, cinnamyl valerate, cognac essential oil, diacetyl, dipropyl ketone, ethyl acetate, ethyl amyl ketone, ethyl butyrate, ethyl cinnamate, ethyl heptanoate, ethyl heptylate, ethyl lactate, ethyl methylphenylglycidate, ethyl nitrate, ethyl propionate, ethyl valerate, heliotropin, hydroxyphenyl-2-butanone (10 percent solution in alcohol), a-ionone, isobutyl anthranilate, isobutyl butyrate, lemon essential oil, maltol, 4-methylacetophenone, methyl anthranilate, methyl benzoate, methyl cinnamate, methyl heptine carbonate, methyl naphthyl ketone, methyl salicylate, mint essential oil, neroli essential oil, nerolin, neryl isobutyrate, orris butter, phenethyl alcohol, rose, rum ether, g-undecalactone, vanillin, and solvent.

I'll be honest and tell you that I have no idea what most of these are. When we eat these foods day in day out, it puts stress on our system. It weakens us. It lowers our immune system. It creates mucus, weight gain, unhappiness, and ageing. Do you want to change? Then you'll need to change the way you feel about these foods.

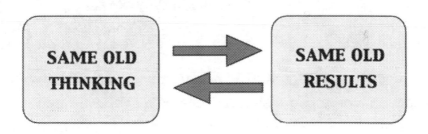

This is serious. "Food" like the milkshake mentioned above isn't food, no matter what the label says. If it is packaged and it has numbers on it, don't eat it. It makes us sick, weak and stressed, and the benefits do not outweigh the repercussions. At the very least, be aware of what you are eating, and limit it to once or twice a month. Meat is another substance that is not a food. Animals are not a food. Just like salt, sugar, canned food, junk food, donuts, chips and fast food, we eat it, but eating animals put stress on our body. Long-term effects are well known. Why put ourselves through that in the first place? Alcohol, coffee, tea, hot chocolate, cola, all soft drinks, mineral water and supermarket fruit juices also put strain on your body.

"Everything in moderation," you might say, but can you see how many unhealthy substances you take, even if it is in moderation? It takes thirty-two glasses of alkaline water to neutralize cola. Everything we eat and drink, our body will try to neutralize it. Coffee dehydrates to the ratio of one to six; that means you need to drink six glasses of water to the one cup of coffee. It is one to four for tea. This does not include the eight glasses of water that we are meant to drink every day. Every food and drink has either a positive effect or a negative effect on us. Be aware of which ones you choose to build your next cells.

> *"My body will not be a tomb for other creatures."*
> *—Leonardo da Vinci*

Cancer can only grow in an acidic body. An alkaline system simply cannot house diseased cells. We think we need salt to make a meal tasty; we think we need sugar to pick us up again at 3:00 p.m. We think we need meat for strength and protein, but all this is not true. Our lower selves will trick us into believing that it is okay for us to drink that coffee in order to do our business first thing in the morning. Well, it's not. It puts stress on our nervous system. Meat putrefies our body, sugar spreads cancer, and salt hardens the arteries and imbalances calcium and potassium in the body. We can easily do without sugar and salt; we can easily do without meat; we can easily do without dairy products. In fact, our bodies will increase in health because of it. We have the ability to live till 120 years of age easily, if we stick to nature's rules. Have foods that are compatible with your body, and you'll never have to see a doctor again.

> "If you only design menus that are essentially junk or fast food, the whole infrastructure supports junk."
>
> —Jamie Oliver

Why should we only eat foods that are compatible? Can we handle never being sick? Can we handle living to between 120 and 150 years old? Doctors are part of our lives; often, they lend a listening ear as well as taking care of our illnesses. Is it possible that doctors know about stressless foods? Why would they promote dairy milk instead of soymilk? Do you think they know about stressful foods, like dairy products, wheat products and meat, and promote it on purpose? Surely not! But it does keep them in a job.

Just in case, let's eat healthier and remember that our doctors never studied nutrition. Why they feel they can advise us on it is beyond me.

> "Today, more than 95% of all chronic disease is caused by food choice, toxic food ingredients, nutritional deficiencies and lack of physical exercise."
>
> —Mike Adams

You don't just learn how to be healthy; you live it. Being healthy is a lifestyle. And you don't just learn truth; you practice it. It also becomes a lifestyle. We all know how to be good people, but what good does it do if we don't practice it? Also, why would we practice being good on the outside if we can't be good on the inside? Do you really think we can eat junk food and practice love on the outside?

I think the idea is that we go forward, improve, change for the better, even though sometimes we fall backwards. At least when we go backwards, we are very aware of it, and we say to ourselves, "We must get back on the right track again." If you have a problem like high cholesterol, it does not mean that you cut down on fried foods; it means you get rid of fried foods completely and you don't touch them again ever! If alcohol is a problem, then cutting down is not a solution. Never drinking alcohol again is going to be the solution to your problem.

We must change. Change is our journey.

"If the doctors of today do not become the nutritionists of tomorrow, then the nutritionists of today will become the doctors of tomorrow."

—Rockefeller Institute of Medicine research

As humans, we have the ability to identify with a situation while observing another person in that situation. For example, you are watching a person biting into a lemon. Does your face scrunch up? Does your mouth fill with saliva?

Your brain has the ability to give you the same response as the person you are observing. The same goes for when you see a child being beaten up by a group of kids; as he is being kicked, you can identify with the physical pain (even if you've never been kicked before). You can also identify with the psychological injustice done to the boy. You can imagine being in that boy's place. Having said that, I think motive often overrides this when identification is not in our own best interest. For example, all the boys in the group know how painful it is to be kicked, but it is their own interest to be and stay in the group. The boys feel safe being in a gang, and there is no way any of the boys would like to be in the place of the boy who's being beaten.

> *"Nobody is so weird others can't identify with them."*
> —*Rebecca Miller*

If you have seen "Blue Eyes, Brown Eyes" you'll know that when an injustice happens, even on a large scale, people don't speak up, because they want to stay safe in their groups, and speaking up doesn't keep them safe. It hurts us to see this happen; it hurts us deep inside, in our very soul, but those who are in power make us turn a blind eye and allow bullying in our society by large companies and governments. An example of this is that there are more than 9.8 million starving people in the world. Fifteen million children die of hunger each year. Even though we all think this is terrible, nothing will change unless we all stand up and make our government share its riches. Our governments do not share their wealth, even when their riches increase every year.

How safe do we feel when we hear that the country is doing well? We don't think, *Let's do with less and share our wealth with the poor people.* Of course we share our wealth on a small scale with the poor of the world, but it is not enough. The world's total military expenditure in 2011 was 1,546,529,200,000 US dollars. Go figure. It is those in power who have the control over what we do, even when we don't agree with it.

> *"Men may not get all they pay for in this world, but they must certainly pay for all they get."*
>
> —*Frederick Douglass*

I feel this also applies to veganism. We can easily identify with the pain of slaughtered animals, because no one really likes the fact that animals are being hurt. Yet there are no official programs in place for us to be educated on the subject to make an objective decision whether to eat meat or not. We are subjected to pretty pictures of cows happily grazing in the paddock who happily "give" us their milk. We see beautiful packaged meat in our supermarkets. We are desensitised because our parents gave meat to us without asking us first, doctors tell us to eat meat for iron; religion justifies eating animals because God created animals for our use. We are not told the whole picture, especially when it comes to how large the carbon footprint is when eating animals. Supermarket produce does not have to state whether an item is vegan or not. Those who choose to be vegan are labelled "weird" or "hippie-ish," "difficult" or "loose cannons."

> *"One-quarter of what you eat keeps you alive. The other three-quarters keeps your doctor alive."*
>
> —*hieroglyph found in an ancient Egyptian tomb*

The vegan lifestyle is a constant struggle for meateaters to accept, and it will remain this way until there are many more vegans who will put the message out there and it becomes widely acceptable to be a vegan in schools, restaurants, shops and hospitals.

Abattoirs

The killing process has quickened its pace over time, because there is such high demand and not enough hours in a day. Fifty-two billion land animals were slaughtered in 2003, and I believe that number to be 55 billion in 2012. This number does not include fish and animals killed in laboratories, fur farms, animal shelters, zoos, marine parks, circuses, sports, hunting, abuse and neglect. If you add all of these together, the total would be 150 billion animals per year.

We would be appalled if we knew how bad abattoirs really were. Did you know that things go wrong eight out of ten times with the slaughter of the animals? Cows are hung up when they are still conscious, and pigs and chickens get boiled alive because they weren't fully stunned. An animal can come back to consciousness if the stunning was too short. In that case, the animal is supposed to be stunned again, but that never happens, because there is no time. This means that they get skinned or boiled alive. In the case of chickens, an electrical charge goes through them which makes them unconscious. It takes up to ten seconds for the chicken to become unconscious. This is the longest and most painful ten seconds of its life. Have you ever touched an electric fence? How quickly did you let go? Imagine having to hold on for ten seconds.

> "Think occasionally of the suffering of which you spare yourself the sight."
>
> —Albert Schweitzer

At this stage, the chickens should be unconscious but not dead. They will then have their throats and major arteries cut by a worker with a knife. Often, the knife misses the arteries, which leaves the bird conscious. This means that some chickens lift their heads in order to avoid the cutting machine, and therefore they are fully conscious when they go into the boiling machine. This happens to 3,121,617 birds per year and this number increases every year. Normally, their heart is still beating and will bleed out for ninety seconds and produce the clean, white meat we recognize as chicken. If the electric shock killed them, they won't bleed, and the meat from these birds turns brown and will be rejected. Yes, the white meat from a chicken is from a chicken that was still alive when she was cut.

> "Nothing more strongly arouses our disgust than cannibalism, yet we make the same impression on Buddhists and vegetarians, for we feed on babies, though not our own."
> —Robert Louis Stevenson

Food animals have a horrific life, starting from birth; they live in cages their whole lives. Cattle and pigs are castrated without numbing. Piglets' teeth are cut or taken out, and their tails are docked, all without painkillers. Chickens have their beaks cut. Did you know that their beak is like our fingertips? It is highly sensitive.

Cattle are branded, and some have their horns ripped out or cut. There is an enormous amount of blood inside those horns, and the process is extremely painful. Another sad thing is that at the end of their lives, cattle are placed in "holding bays" at or near the abattoir, where they could stay for months. They get fed, but they have to stand in their own filth. They cannot lie down, as they do not lie in their own crap. There is no protection from the weather. In summer, they stand in the heat of the sun, day in day out, and there is no shelter to protect them from the winter months. These animals are gentle, are good mothers, are intelligent and all have their own personalities.

We must know where our food comes from, we must know what suffering animal beings go through, but most of all, we must tell our children about this process if you are an animal eater with children.

> "The reason people awaken is because they have finally stopped agreeing to the things that insult their soul."
> —Anonymous

If you are not ashamed of eating meat, then why not tell your children about it? Go on, answer that question. If you are not ashamed about eating animal beings, why are you not telling your children how it came to be on their plate? Why not take them to an abattoir? Could it be you want to protect your child from this horror? Could it be that children are so pure, with pure souls we don't want to taint with the cruelty of animal eating? Could it be that eating animal beings is such a normal occurrence in our lives, and we just give it to them, and by the time they find out what it is, they won't think twice about it?

But who are you kidding? If you feel any awkwardness or guilt about your own meat-eating habits, how could you give meat to your child, who believes you would only do the best thing for him and you would never do anything to harm him? Why not keep eating animal beings for yourself but not give it to your child until he is old enough to decide for himself to eat death or not? Nothing is going to happen to your child if he doesn't eat flesh; in fact, he will be healthier for it.

> *"I became a vegetarian after realizing that animals feel afraid, cold, hungry and unhappy like we do."*
>
> —Cesar Chavez

Was this last paragraph uncomfortable for you? Well, think about how uncomfortable food animals are, right now, this day, every day until their horrific and painstaking death, just so you can have something to put into your mouth. Think about it.

> *"We cut the throat of a calf and hang it up by the heels to bleed to death so that our veal cutlet may be white; we nail geese to a board and cram them with food because we like the taste of liver disease; we tear birds to pieces to decorate our women's hats; we mutilate domestic animals for no reason at all except to follow an instinctively cruel fashion; and we connive at the most abominable tortures in the hope of discovering some magical cure for our own diseases by them."*
>
> —George Bernard Shaw

Raw Food

Even though I eat a lot of raw food, I am not an advocate for a completely raw-food diet. I love my cooked food, the soups, the stews, rice dishes, etc. I do, however, never boil my food or let the temperatures go above 40 degrees. Nearly all minerals and most vitamins are destroyed by heat. Steaming is just as bad, and microwaved food is foodless food. If you must soften your food, then use as little water as possible, and then drink the water or use it in your stew or soups. Heat it up in as little time as possible, and eat the veggies straight away. The longer our fruit and veggies are exposed to light and oxygen, the more nutritional loss there is.

Please, never cook or heat up food in the microwave oven. Get out of the habit. There are many studies that prove nutritional loss, carcinogenic properties, and an overall fall in immune potential. Educate yourself on this subject.

We must eat at least 60 percent of our food raw. If we don't eat raw food, as we get older, we'll lose the ability to digest raw food. When this happens, doctors will advise us to blanche our food, which makes our veggies easier to digest. How sad is it when we can no longer digest broccoli, cauliflower and tofu just because we never had it in its original state. Raw food is the only thing that will give us the enzymes to digest raw food! Please encourage your children to eat raw foods like carrots and salads with raw cauliflower and broccoli. Never peel your foods either. If your child gags on a apple peel, he'll work it out. Do not bend towards your child's demands for peeled carrots. If you don't make a fuss, then that behaviour will go away. Also, it's okay for your child to eat watermelon pips. You must eat them as well, as they are the most nutritional part of the watermelon. How sad it is that we now buy fruits that are missing their seeds. Grapes, apples, bananas, lemons, cucumbers and watermelon all are modified to have fewer seeds. Seeds are the lungs of a fruit. It is the very ingredient that makes a fruit healthy. The more seeds a fruit has, the healthier it is for you.

> *"The food you eat can either be the safest and most powerful form of medicine or the slowest form of poison."*
>
> —Anne Wigmore

We must have our raw greens, and one way to do this is is to prepare them into a grand salad. Include beans, sprouts, shredded carrots, shredded beetroot, nuts and seeds. Any nuts and seeds that you use should be soaked in water and a little apple-cider vinegar overnight or at the very least a few hours before you eat them. This will activate the seed ready for sprouting. It is a wonderful way for us to have alive foods. Of course, include parsley and celery, capsicum, home-grown tomatoes, cucumber and sliced zucchini in your salad. The lettuce should be dark green or red. Even though iceberg lettuce is a favourite, it is acidic, and only the outer dark-green leaves should be used. I'm not a big fan of dressings, as they are extremely acidic and will undo any good the salad will do to our body, so get out of the habit of using any kind of dressings. The other day, I was given a dressing of carrot juice and tahini and tamari. It was very nice, and for those who need dressing, this is a good alternative. Please try to have the salad in its organic state; no salt or pepper required. Do not mix fruit into your green salad; keep the two separate. I'm also not a fan of mushrooms, because they were not grown in the sun. I do believe that if you eat mushrooms from your field in season, that is fine, but otherwise it is a burden on your body, and you'll feel sleepy after your meal. That is actually a really good way to know if a food is a burden on your body or not. If your body needs too much energy to digest it, we will feel tired soon afterwards.

I don't believe in food that putrefies the body. Have leeks instead of onions. Leeks contain chlorophyll, which onions don't have. Chlorophyll is the life-blood force of plants. It is the very thing that gives a plant its green colour. Only have garlic when you are sick or have worms. Garlic is medicinal. I think April in the Southern Hemisphere and September in the Northern Hemisphere is a great time to have a "garlic boost" to boost your immunity before winter. This is what you do to prepare this boost, peel whole garlic cloves and soften them in a little water in a saucepan over low heat, but don't boil them. Once the cloves have softened and cooled, eat them directly, and use the liquid in soup or stew. I recommend consuming four cloves twice per day for three to four days, and the whole family can get a boost. However, choose the days when you prepare this carefully, as it's smelly, but it's well worth it.

> "And, most dear actors, eat no onions nor garlic, for we are to utter sweet breath."
>
> —William Shakespeare (1564–1616)
> A Midsummer Night's Dream

Dairy Products

Yes, the time has come to talk about this gruesome subject that brings so much suffering to animals in one way and more so to the environment and human health in another way. You vegetarians thought you would get away with just being a vegetarian. No, I am here to convert you. This section is for you especially. Being a vegetarian instead of a vegan is like being a religious nut who doesn't go to church or a health nut who only eats organic chips. Get the point? Ask yourself why you haven't gone the whole way.

I'll start with the most basic question asked when people find out I do not consume any dairy: Where do you get your calcium? Really? I find it hard not to be rude to people when they ask me that question. I start by saying, "Well, the same way all mammals get their calcium... by eating their greens." We also get plenty of calcium from herbs, tahini, tofu, seeds and nuts, beans, broccoli and lemons. It is hard not to get calcium.

> *"There is no 'need' for us to eat meat, dairy or eggs. Indeed, these foods are increasingly linked to various human diseases and animal agriculture is an environmental disaster for the planet."*
>
> *—Gary L. Francione*

Take a moment and think of a cow. This is a strong animal that signifies a classic "calcium mammal," compared to a "sodium mammal" like a goat. Think about the differences between the two mammals. A cow eats primarily grass, is stiff and walks around the place. A goat eats everything in its path; it climbs, it jumps, it's fast on its feet, plays and is flexible. Goats thrive where a cow would starve to death. Goats are browsers, living on bushes, leaves, bark and grass, whereas the cow is a grazer, sticking to the ground. Out of the two animals, which do you think a human mammal identifies with more? We are also sodium mammals. If we drink the milk from a calcium mammal, then we become like them. We become stiff and slow, our nails start hardening, and we age. Cow's milk contains a larger percentage of salts for the purpose of forming horns, hooves, hide and large bones. Human and goat milk is made up of more sulphur, chlorine and potassium.

I do not believe we should drink any animal milk unless it is human mother's milk. It will not produce catarrh, phlegm and mucus like cow's milk does.

> "Every time you drink a glass of milk or eat a piece of cheese, you harm a mother. Please go vegan."
> —Gary L. Francione

Osteoporosis—The next question I usually get asked is: what about the risk of getting osteoporosis? Osteoporosis is a condition that makes our bones fragile. What makes them fragile in the first place is the loss of calcium. The one thing that leaches calcium out of our bones more than anything else is animal protein. Yes! Meat, eggs, seafood and dairy all take calcium out of your bones and cause osteoporosis. Proteins from plant-based products do not leach calcium out of our bones. The Osteoporosis Foundation does not think so and says it needs further studies. Let's look further. Let's look at who suffers rampant osteoporosis the most. Caucasians and Eskimos are on top of the list, and they generally consume one thousand to two thousand milligrams of calcium daily, compared to Australian Aboriginals, Amazon tribes and Bantu women, who consume around two hundred milligrams per day and rarely get osteoporosis. The Australian recommended daily allowance is between one thousand and thirteen hundred milligrams.

Every six minutes, someone is admitted to hospital for an osteoporosis fracture, right now here in Australia. That will rise to every three to four minutes in 2021, according to the Osteoporosis Australia Medical & Scientific Advisory Committee. A Harvard University study done by the Physicians Committee found that women who drank the most cow's milk also suffered the most bone fractures! This twelve-year Harvard Nurses' Health Study found that those who consumed the most calcium from dairy foods broke more bones than those who rarely drank milk. This was a broad study based on 77,761 women aged 34 through 59.After consuming animal protein, the next time we urinate it is full of calcium which has been leached from our bones and that is how we lose it. (3)

If you want to promote healthy bones, then your own organic vegetable juice is on top of my list, together with exercise and sunlight. Eat soy products, as they contain estrogens which keep bones strong.

"Consumption of dairy products, particularly at age 20 years, was associated with an increased risk of hip fracture in old age."

—"Case-Control Study of Risk Factors for Hip Fractures in the Elderly." American Journal of Epidemiology, *Vol. 139, No. 5, 1994.*

No coffee or tea, no alcohol or smoking, salt, sugar or chocolate. Check out your medications, as a lot of them also increase the chance of osteoporosis, like HRT, corticosteroids, antidepressants, blood thinners, Methotrexate, thyroid hormones and some drugs used for epilepsy.

The Horrors of the Dairy Industry—A young cow of about eighteen months is artificially inseminated for the first time. A heifer will be pregnant for seven to nine months before she is induced, in order to have the calf in a short period of time. A national survey shows that the practice of induction is declining, but we really don't know how widespread the practice is.

The calf is taken away within a twelve- to twenty-four-hour period, and the commercial milking process has begun. She is highly strung at this point, clearly showing stress and suffering, as she has been separated from her calf. Cows are extremely good mothers and will defend their babies with all their might. They will cry for weeks. Apart from the emotional pain, there is also the physical pain. Calves naturally will suckle off and on throughout the whole day, just like our human babies. It means that our boobs don't fill up too much over time, because that is very painful. Well, this new heifer mum will be relieved only twice per day. Her udder becomes huge and very painful. She'll end up giving ten times more milk every day than she would naturally with her calf. The cow's teats become infected, and pus and blood are commonly found in milk.

> "I became vegan because I saw footage of what really goes on in the slaughterhouses and on the dairy farms."
> —Ellen DeGeneres

That is not all that is found in milk. There is faeces, bacteria, antibiotics, pesticides and hormones found in every glass of milk that you drink.

Most of the protein in milk is casein. Casein is used to make many plastic products, paints and glues. Casein binds together anything from furniture to processed foods. People are often allergic to casein, and it produces mucus in our system, as our body finds it hard to dispose of.

The food that this heifer is given is *all* genetically modified. The grain she is fed is unnatural, and this puts immense strain on her digestive system. All the food that intensively farmed Australian animals eat is genetically modified. If you do not want to eat GM food, then do not eat animals! If you do, then you have ingested a GM product. Cheese is even worse. It takes ten pounds of milk to make one pound of cheese.

> *Calves are taken from their mother 12 – 24 hours after birth. Research has shown that there is a strong maternal bond between a mother cow and her calf. Mother cows show strong signs of grieving after their calf is removed and will bellow desperately for it to return.*
>
> *Animals Australia – The voice for animals.*

The new heifer mum will be inseminated again about two months later, and the whole process continues until she is about seven years old, and then she is off to the slaughterhouse. Often, these dairy cows are so weak and diseased that they can hardly walk up to the slaughterhouse, and they are beaten, kicked, and poked with electric probes. What a horrible life for this beautiful, gentle mother who is intelligent and has great memory.

Now, what about her calves? If it is a "heifer calf," then she'll still be taken away and weaned off the milk. About one quarter of all heifer calves will become replacements for their mums. The other three quarters and almost all bull calves will be taken for veal production. They feed them milk replacer, but not often, because they'll go to the slaughterhouse within being five days old. The milk replacement is very low in iron, which makes the calf anaemic, and this gives the meat that pinkish colour. They spend the entire time in crates which are 60 centimetres wide and 1.8 metres long. Some calves will live in these crates for up to twenty-three weeks. These babies cannot walk, as their muscles are extremely weak. The caretaker of these calves will put a collar around their necks which is attached to a chain hanging from the ceiling. This stops the calf from lying down, because the chain hangs as low as the calf's head, forcing it to stand up its whole life. The reason why the calf is not allowed to lie down is because it could never get up again. Other dairy farms have an incinerator near the birthing stall and the calves are thrown in straight after birth… alive.

At least eight hundred thousand calves in Australia are slaughtered every year, and because they are a by-product rather than having any value, they are treated extremely badly. For the few bobby calves that are raised to become steers, this also leads to a life of misery and pain. Tail-docking is still legal, and so is dehorning or horn-trimming, branding as well as castration. All these procedures are done without the use of anaesthetics.

There are 29 million cattle in Australia, 9 million of which will be slaughtered every year. There are 2.01 million dairy cows in Australia, giving the consumer 10.125 billion litres of milk every year. Each cow will produce five thousand litres of milk. That averages out to each person drinking 103 litres of milk per year and eating 13 kilos of cheese per year. All these cows eat and drink a lot. Each cow eats about 40 kilos of food a day, and dairy cows drink up to 190 litres every day. Beef cattle will drink about one hundred litres of water every day.

> *"In a world where people 'milk' animals for every last penny they can make out of them, cows drew the short straw. Cows are some of the most interesting and social animals, with a world of emotions that could be likened to our own, yet we take their babies, their milk, their freedom, their skin, their life ..."*
>
> *—Animals Australia*

The food grown to feed these animals could feed 8.7 million people. Cows also produce a lot of manure, which pollutes waterways and soils. One cow produces as much as 120 pounds of manure every day, which is the same as what over 30 people produce every day. The animal methane which is expelled has seventy-two times more impact on our environment than CO_2 pollution, which is a lot more than what is generated by coal-fired power stations. Cows tend to do a dump when they are being milked, and every time "milking time" has finished, the farmer has to clean his milking plant thoroughly. Enormous amounts of water and chemicals are used twice every day. There are 9,256 dairy farms in Australia, and an average dairy farm will use 47 million litres of water every year.

If you think that is a lot of water, think about this: for every kilo of steak, it can take up to fifty thousand litres of water to produce it. The dairy and beef industry has a huge impact on our environment, as this industry alone contributes over 30 percent to global greenhouse gas emissions. The equivalent to one litre of milk is to drive twenty kilometres in a car. The CSIRO (Commonwealth Scientific and Industrial Research Organisation) and the University of Adelaide estimated that farmed animals are responsible for 92 percent of land degradation.

> "There is no 'need' for us to eat meat, dairy or eggs. Indeed, these foods are increasingly linked to various human diseases and animal agriculture is an environmental disaster for the planet."
>
> —Gary L. Francione

So, for those vegetarians who care about our environment, this should be enough reason never to touch dairy again. For those vegetarians who care about their health, you will be so much healthier without dairy. For those who are vegetarians because they care about animals, please understand the cruelty that happens in this industry; and for those vegetarians who are apathetic towards this subject, ask yourself why and ask yourself: "Where else in life am I apathetic?"

Allergies

Asthma, arthritis, eczema, sinus and hay fever all have one similarity—they are all caused by an overload of toxins in the body from consuming the wrong foods and drinks over a period of time. Today, there is way too much food in the Western world. Unfortunately, 95 percent of it is the wrong kind of food, and our systems cannot get rid of the toxins fast enough. This results in toxin overload. People are overweight and this gives a clear indication that the person suffers from malnutrition. Did you know that there are now more overweight people in the world than there are starving people in third-world countries?

Eating the wrong foods lowers our immunity. With an underactive immune system, our bodies are too tired to function properly, and instead of us throwing out rubbish, our bodies just accumulate and accumulate rubbish. Of course, a person can be allergic to the substances in the air, such as pollens, pollutants, dust and animal hair, but it is the efficiency with which our bodies deal with this that gives us a clue of how healthy we are.

For example: I am extremely allergic to dust, and twice a year, I get challenged with this allergy when I swap my summer clothes over for my winter clothes and vice versa. Within twenty minutes, I will start to sneeze, as a lot of mucus comes up through my bronchials and sinuses. My immune system gets activated, and my body will begin to make antibodies naturally. This swapping over does not take longer than half an hour, and as soon as it is over, I wash my hands and face and eat something with high vitamin content, and it is over straight away.

This is my immune system working perfectly. If I want to be hard on myself, I would say, "Well, if my system was totally clean and my immunity was at 100 percent, then I wouldn't be allergic at all," and I would be quite correct in saying that. This is the same for every person who suffers from hay fever, dust or anything they are allergic to that floats in the air. I cringe when people go to doctors for this and they prescribe antihistamines, decongestants and steroids. These medications push the problem deeper into your system and give the brain a message to ignore the allergy. That's why it stops—not because the problem was resolved but because the brain was forced to ignore it. Why doesn't the doctor tell the person to increase his immunity by increasing vitamin content and stop eating the wrong foods which caused the allergic reaction in the first place?

"By cleansing your body on a regular basis and eliminating as many toxins as possible from your environment, your body can begin to heal itself, prevent disease, and become stronger and more resilient than you ever dreamed possible!"
—Dr. Edward Group III

Seventy-eight percent of Aussies have experienced allergies. That is a lot, and the figures point towards increase. If medication helps, why is there an increase? Why did we not experience these allergies fifty years ago? Anyone over the age of forty never even heard of allergies like today, especially allergies towards peanuts. A hundred years ago, asthma did not even exist.

Just how much have allergies and asthma grown? Figures from the World Allergy Organization reveal the global prevalence of asthma has increased by an astounding 50 percent every decade for the past forty years, and peanut allergies have tripled since 1997.

Scientists are frantically working on a cure for allergies. Why? Why not work out what caused them in the first place? Like too many sugars, too many fats, too much junk food, soft drinks, alcohol, coffee, tea, and too many wheat products. It really isn't difficult to work out why they never had allergies forty years ago: they didn't have the amount of junk food back then. Allergies costs the Australian economy between 7.8 and 11.2 billion dollars every year.

> "We got so much food in America we're allergic to food. Allergic to food! Hungry people ain't allergic to shit. You think anyone in Rwanda's got a f*cking lactose intolerance?!"
> —Chris Rock

Any catarrhal discharge is a symptom of an allergy and toxicity overload. Because the bowel finds it difficult to digest the mucus, we find that allergy and asthma patients also have underactive bowels. The wrong foods are acidic, and this irritates the stomach and forms a membrane of mucus. Alkaline foods will neutralize the stomach and stop the irritation; eating lots of greens will stimulate the stomach again. The healing process is very simple.

Eczema and psoriasis are skin disorders, and the number of people diagnosed increases every year. The cause of this is an overload of acidic foods over a long period of time. The way to solve it is to have alkaline foods and drinks and do a detox and never eat junk food again. Green powders like chlorella, spirulina, wheatgrass and liquid chlorophyll are extremely good for people with this condition, and all will be cleared up within two weeks of committing to a better diet. Again in this case, the bowel is very acidic and needs to return to alkaline.

Today, there are 9 million Australians who have asthma. Asthma stems from too much mucus build-up from dairy foods, wheat products and other acidic foods. Bronchitis and asthma are just a way for our bodies to eliminate mucus. You must never stop this process. Please change your diet, and you will never have to have asthma or bronchitis again. It is that simple!

Okay, let's look at arthritis. Again, this condition is 100 percent caused by the foods we eat. Rheumatism and any stiff and painful joints are the result of inflammation caused by acidic foods. Our stomach wall needs alkalinity, and organic green sodium is the element that keeps it soft and healthy. The minute we eat acidic food, the sodium is destroyed, and our body takes the sodium which is stored in our joints to compensate and directs it to our stomach wall to keep it soft and healthy as long as possible. What happens is that sodium keeps the calcium in our joints flexible, and when that is removed, the calcium becomes stiff. So, all we have to do is eat lots of sodium foods like spinach, green-leafed vegetables, dulse, okra, parsley, celery, organic veggie juices and alkaline fruits high in vitamin C like kiwifruit, to bring back the sodium in our joints again, which is our sodium reserve.

Please understand that I am *not* talking about salt. Salt is not a food but a preservative, which our bodies have a lot of problems dealing with.

> *"Chronic indigestion, intestinal irritation, constipation, ulcers and other stomach disorders as well as joint troubles such as arthritis, rheumatism and osteoporosis are often signs that the bio-organic sodium is deficient in the body."*
>
> *—Dr. Bernard Jensen*

So, how simple is that? It is not easy to stick to, but it is worth it. How are you going to remember what to eat or not, which foods are good foods or not?

This is how I do my check: would a gorilla in the wild eat it? If the answer is no, then don't eat it. You will never see a gorilla with allergies or arthritis, because he doesn't eat the foods that cause it. Interestingly, when gorillas are in captivity and eat our foods, they do get sick and suffer from the same conditions as we do.

A gorilla is a vegan. Every now and then, it will eat ants, but that is no more than twice per year. Every other meal is leaves, grasses, nuts and seeds, fruits and vegetables. Does a gorilla in the wild eat ice cream? No, he doesn't, and so you shouldn't. Does he eat chips, meat, donuts? No, so neither should you. Of course, we can be more flexible than that. Our health is built on what we eat most days, and it is okay to have junk every now and then, because it is what we do every day that matters. Make sure that at least 70 percent of your food and drinks are alkaline, and you will be all right. You cannot eat animal proteins if you want to be healthy, because animal protein causes us to be in a constant state of inflammation. Read that last sentence again. Animal protein causes the body to be in a constant state of inflammation.

Sandra's Super Foods

These foods are immunity strengtheners. Include these foods in your everyday life. They are not presented in any order, and not all of them are essential at the same time, but I do encourage you to try them all and see which ones benefit you the most. Make the decision to be healthier not at home, but at the supermarket. Start by not bringing junk food into your home in the first place. Grow your own food as much as possible; find a way. If you can, please buy organically grown food, and also buy from the farmers' markets. Yes, it is more expensive, but because you are not buying any more junk, this money can now go towards health foods.

Water has to be on top of my list. Our planet, like our bodies, consists of 75 percent water. Water is teeming with interdimensional life. Water feeds the cells of all living things and helps to build cartilage and bones. We can use water to heal ourselves and eliminate toxins. Did you know that often, when we are thirsty, our brains will signal that we are hungry, since natural foods also have a high water content? Drinking water will change our appetite; it fills you up, and you can lose weight just by drinking lots of water.

> "The doctor of the future will no longer treat the human frame with drugs, but rather will cure and prevent disease with nutrition."
>
> —Thomas Edison

Liquid chlorophyll is the greatest blood cleanser and blood builder. You put this green liquid in your water. Give it to your kids. It gives you perfect stools, as it alkalises your system. Get into the habit that every time you drink water, you squirt a little chlorophyll into it.

Chlorella—I could write a whole chapter on the benefits of chlorella, but I'll just give you some information about this super food. Please consume this in powder form in a glass of water. Get over the smell and taste; just do it. Powder is far more easily absorbed than tablets. Chlorella is a complete protein, with very high vitamin B12 benefits. Please always buy organically grown chlorella. Synergy and Melrose both sell a fantastic chlorella product.

Spirulina—This super food contains over one hundred nutrients, and this you also consume in powder form with water. Synergy and Melrose both sell these products.

Barley and wheatgrass powder: these are 100 percent alkaline foods. This food has nothing to do with whether you are allergic to wheat or not, as the powder is made from the greens and not the seeds.

What I tend to do is put a small amount of my chlorella, spirulina, barley and wheatgrass powders together in a dark jar, mix it well, and have a teaspoon of this powder every day. Please note that light and oxygen kills any goodness, so as soon as you pour water into the glass with the powder, drink it.

Maca powder: Maca is a native plant that grows in the Andes of Peru, and its root is highly nutritious. I found that this super food gave me stamina. I have it every morning in my banana milkshake. You can find the recipe on page 243. Bonvit makes this product.

Unhulled tahini—This super food makes us strong. It promotes health on all levels. Please only buy the unhulled tahini and use it in shakes and instead of butter and peanut butter. Have a tablespoon by itself. Tahini has a higher concentration of calcium than any other food.

Alive foods like sprouted seeds, alfalfa, bean, radish, broccoli, sunflower, green-leaf sprouts and all other sprouted versions are all extremely rich in antioxidants. Use them in your salads, sandwiches; a handful per day should do for excellent health. Please educate yourself on this subject. You can learn how to sprout at home and then use different varieties of seeds that you would like to sprout.

Berries—all berries, are super foods, and we should eat them for their antioxidants, high vitamin content, cancer-fighting properties, anti-aging and high-fibre benefits. Organic blueberries have to be up there, blackberries, goji, acai, bilberries, gooseberries, strawberries, raspberries, elderberries and cranberries are all super foods. Eat the ones in season, and try to grow some of them. Eat some every day, but you don't need much. Eat them by themselves, and never have them in yogurt.

Avocado—Avocados are one of the best anti-ageing super foods to have. Always include avocados in salads, use them for spreads, or eat them just the way they are.

Nuts and Seeds—Oh my goodness, these are so important in our everyday diet. Nuts contain powerful anti-inflammatories, and heart disease is an inflammatory condition. Almonds and other nuts need to be activated before eating. This means you soak them in water overnight and they plump up. Wash all seeds and nuts before eating them. Walnut is an important nut for the brain, but I really am in favour of all nuts and seeds. Please use a large variety of them in their natural form and not salted. Some people like to soak nuts in Apple cider vinegar. The reason is that no bacteria can grow in Apple cider vinegar.

Beetroot is my favourite super vegetable and should be eaten every day. It is a blood-builder. It is high in iron and vitamin C. Have it raw, grated in your salads and wraps. Have it in your juices with carrot and celery. Try growing your own beetroot. It is very easy, and you can use the leaves in your salad and juices. These leaves have more iron than spinach leaves. You can steam the beetroot leaves like you would spinach. Please note that it will turn your urine and stools red.

Broccoli has some amazing properties and should be eaten every day, raw in salads or lightly steamed. You can eat the stems and the leaves as well and include them in soups and stir-fries.

Spinach is a very important vegetable. Have it in salads, soups, stir-fries and juices. Make spinach a part of your everyday diet.

Organic Soy, Tofu and Tempeh—Please note that I wrote "organic." If any soy product is not organic, then don't buy it, because it will be genetically modified. In Australia, we are really lucky with the high standard of soy products. Soy products have phytoestrogens, which have oestrogen-like qualities. These substances seem to be associated with a lower risk of breast, prostate and colon cancer and reduced incidence of heart disease, as well as osteoporosis. Soy is a complete protein, and it contains vitamins B and E, choline, iron, potassium and phosphorus.

Green Juices—When we need to increase our immunity, if we want to detox, and when we are not well, we really need to have juices far above everything else. I find carrot, celery, beetroot, kale and parsley a must. You can include everything that is growing in your garden at the moment. I think cucumber is always wonderful, and capsicum and spinach are all favourable. Please do not include fruits with this; the two do not go together because of the high sugar in fruits.

Organic Watermelon—I must stress that you eat organic watermelon with the pips. Eat it by itself or juice it by itself, and your body will get a wonderful cleanse.

Fruits—Apples, bananas, dragonfruit, red grapes with seeds, pomegranate, avocado, black currants, cranberry mangosteen, goji, strawberries, figs and raspberries. Please only buy organic fruit or grow your own.

Coconut Oil—This oil can be heated to very high temperatures without changing. Please educate yourself on the benefits of coconut oil.

Food Pyramid: We are all familiar with the standard food pyramid, which was developed by Harvard University as a guide for what to eat. Dieticians are still modifying it all the time as new statistics show how bad animal proteins and wheat products are for us.

Below is a pyramid that I feel is the most accurate. Tofu belongs in the protein area, and I would add coconut oil to the oils and take out the yeast.

I think if you use this pyramid as a guide, you'll do well. Please drink lots of water every day and exercise at least twenty minutes three times per week. Adults and children should be physically active every day for at least an hour.

The Raw Food Pyramid

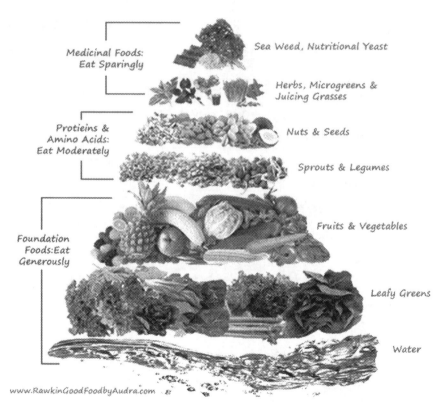

Medicinal Foods:
Eat Sparingly

Sea Weed, Nutritional Yeast

Herbs, Microgreens &
Juicing Grasses

Protieins &
Amino Acids:
Eat Moderately

Nuts & Seeds

Sprouts & Legumes

Foundation
Foods:Eat
Generously

Fruits & Vegetables

Leafy Greens

Water

www.RawkinGoodFoodbyAudra.com

Kids' Lunchbox Fillers

I would start as early as possible with feeding your child a clean diet. There is absolutely no reason why children need fats and sugars in their lunchboxes. Include foods that are in season; for example, when asparagus is in season, include some raw asparagus in the lunchbox, and please do not peel the skin—or any skin of any food, for that matter.

Here are some suggestions for your kids' lunchbox, taken from a week of my own kids' lunchboxes.

Monday—Grapes, cucumber strips, carrot sticks, mandarin, sunflower seeds, two nori sheets and a bottle of water with chlorophyll.

Tuesday—Apple, grapes, carrot sticks, mandarin, banana, selection of seeds and nuts, two nori sheets and a bottle of water with chlorophyll.

Wednesday—Nori or sushi rolls (brown rice with yummy filling like avocado, cucumber and grated carrot), apple, mandarin, grapes and bottle of water with chlorophyll.

Thursday—Two dolmades, cantaloupe, nuts and seed mixture, apple, banana, two nori sheets and a bottle of water with chlorophyll.

Friday—A wrap with leftover salad from the night before as filling, grapes, fruit cup, kiwifruit and a bottle of water with chlorophyll.

> "We cannot solve the problems with the same thinking that created them."
>
> —Albert Einstein

As apples go out of season, stone fruits appear. When the weather gets colder, citrus fruits come into season. This is the only time of the year we eat citrus, and preferably it is from our own or our neighbour's trees.

We'll include passionfruits, strawberries, blueberries, watermelon and celery sticks in their lunchboxes.

Rice-paper rolls are always a favourite. Often we'll have them on a Sunday, and we'll make some extra for Monday's school lunch. The same goes for salads throughout the week; we always make enough for the next day's lunchboxes.

> "Then God said, 'I give you every seed-bearing plant on the face of the whole earth and every tree that has fruit with seed in it. They will be yours for food. And to all the beasts of the earth and all the birds of the air and all the creatures that move on the ground—everything that has the breath of life in it—I give every green plant for food.'"
>
> —Genesis 1:29–30

Saturday and Sunday, we eat what we like, but during the week, we eat our dinner at the table, and it is always four to five vegetables, tofu or some other vegetarian protein and salad. We have big meals, and our variety is large, but everything we eat is easy to digest.

We break this up with stews, soups, rice dishes, polenta and couscous dishes. One thing I like to note is that I do not like eating nightshade plants twice in a row. Three times per week is plenty, and less is even better.

Nightshades are a group of foods that have compounds in them we call alkaloids. I could go into great detail explaining what that is, but in simple terms, it contributes to joint inflammation. If you have joint problems, osteoarthritis, rheumatoid arthritis or gout, I would minimize eating nightshades. They include potatoes, tomatoes, capsicums, eggplants and paprika.

Please keep pasta to a minimum. It is glue with an acidic sauce. I love the spaghetti plant, and that can be a substitute for real spaghetti.

One thing that might surprise people is that I feed my dog only vegan food. It didn't make sense to me to fight for animal rights and then have my dog indulge in food from this cruel industry. Our dog was two and a half when we got her from the pound, and she had been raised on meat. She had itchy skin, which was very annoying for her. She would bite the areas around her legs until they were red and raw. Not long after I put her on a vegan diet, she stopped being itchy. She became calmer, and her coat became thick and shiny. She is now nearly nine years old and extremely healthy. I do not believe she is missing out on anything; in fact, she loves her food.

This is what I give her to eat: I take my big soup pot and cook rice, lentils, beans or any kind of legumes that I happen to have. It is time to include the veggies when this has cooked. I put all kinds of vegetables in a blender, and when it is small, I put it in the big soup pot with the cooked rice (or whatever). I stir it and put in my herbs and salt or vegan gravy. I fry tofu cubes which have been sautéed in soy sauce. I stir them in and cook until veggies are soft. I freeze the dog food in take-away containers. Play around with this, as different dogs like different things. Also look on the Web for recipes.

"Many people are surprised to learn that not only can dogs enjoy vibrant health on a vegan diet, but just like people, their physical condition can actually improve as a result of eliminating animal foods."

—Gentle World

Rainbow Salad

What a lovely name for a salad! What it basically means is that we include all the different foods with different colours. Did you know that each colour has its own vibration? Well, each food with its own different colour also has its own nutritional vibration. Colour is very important to us, as it attracts us to different fruits and vegetables. We can see seven major colours in the rainbow. They are the same colours as our chakras: red, orange, yellow, green, blue, indigo and violet.

Red—This is a stimulant. Red foods like beetroot, red cabbage, tomatoes, strawberries and red capsicum will stimulate a person physically, mentally and spiritually. This colour brings out emotions and should be used when vitality is low and when blood circulation is poor.

Orange—Foods that are orange stimulate creativity and ambition through energetic activity. Too much orange fruit like oranges can produce great nervousness and restless behaviour. Pumpkin is a great orange food to put into our rainbow salad. Fry little cubes of pumpkin in coconut oil until brown and then sprinkle some tamari or soy sauce on it, and this will coat the cubes. This tastes great in the salad.

Yellow—Yellow fruits and vegetables tend to be laxative to the bowel and calming to the nerves. These include corn, yellow tomatoes, yellow capsicum, pineapples, peaches, bananas, mangoes and squash. Yellow is a joyful colour, and it also brings out wisdom and understanding. It is a great colour in the kitchen.

Green—This colour stimulates generosity on a mental plane and elimination on a physical plane. What a great colour. Its foods represent soothing and healing, allowing our body to rejuvenate. Here are some foods perfect for our rainbow salad: avocado, asparagus, broccoli, celery, cucumber, kale, green-leafed lettuce, rocket, brussels sprouts (finely cut up), zucchini, peas and green beans.

Blue—This is a slowing-down colour. There are no true blue vegetables, but I think blue beans, blue cabbage and blue potatoes come close. You can use the blue beans and cabbage in your salad. Blueberries is the obvious blue fruit, but I would not recommend putting fruit into a salad.

> "The first gatherings of the garden in May of salads, radishes and herbs made me feel like a mother about her baby—how could anything so beautiful be mine. And this emotion of wonder filled me for each vegetable as it was gathered every year. There is nothing that is comparable to it, as satisfactory or as thrilling, as gathering the vegetables one has grown.
> —Alice B. Toklas

Indigo—These foods stimulate inner growth. It represents the breakthrough point, where problems are seen as stepping stones to wonderful solutions. Foods with this colour are:

purple grapes, plums, cherries, raisins, indigo cauliflower, purple onions, blackberries, acai berries and eggplant. When you use eggplant in your salad, use the same preparation as with pumpkin: cut it all up in cubes, and fry it in coconut oil until browned.

Violet—This is the greatest healing colour; it represents the highest motives and spiritual aspirations. When we eat these foods, the body, soul and spirit are harmonised and energised. These foods include: purple basil, purple capsicum, kohlrabi, black tomatoes, dulse, elderberries, passionfruit and wild rice.

So these are the foods you can use to make a Rainbow Salad. Please do not use dressing. Learn to enjoy your salad as it is. Salad should be eaten at the end of dinner. Eat salad instead of dessert. Please get out of the habit of eating dessert.

Bread—Bread is responsible for fatigue, bloating and headaches. Bread turns into sugar and causes blood-sugar levels to rise, which stops the burning up of fat. This is just a small problem compared to the rest. Bread is baked incredibly fast and at very high temperatures. This process is possible because of the high amounts of yeast, additives, stabilisers and preservatives and also gives it extremely long shelf life. Some researchers believe this could help fuel diabetes. A study by the Cancer Council of Australia, which followed more than thirty-six thousand people for four years, found those who ate the most white bread were more than 30 percent more likely to develop type-2 diabetes.

Personally, I think if you eat live breads like Ezekiel or Organic sprouted bread every now and then, it is okay. Have a look at the ingredients in supermarket bread, and compare it to healthier bread; you'll be astounded. Keep bread to a minimum, because usually what we spread on it isn't that good for us either. Better to have organic wholemeal wraps with salad in them.

The perfect sandwich: Take green lettuce, avocado, cucumber, organic tomato, capsicum, a little raw onion, herbs such as basil, coriander and parsley, and put all this together. Now ditch the bread and eat the rest.

> *"For all things produced in a garden, whether of salads or fruits, a poor man will eat better that has one of his own, than a rich man that has none."*
>
> —J.C. Loudoun

General Well-Being—The chemistry of man is affected by physical, mental, and spiritual attributes, and when these are working in harmony, the life force lifts our health level and brings us back to a state of wellness. People need to be taught how to live, and knowing how to live, they'll outgrow the need for a doctor. This is what they need to learn:

1. Every disease is a result of wrong living habits.
2. "Dis-ease" will automatically leave the body when the person knows the "art of living correctly."
3. Nature always works towards perfect health.
4. Each person's sickness depends on the way he disobeyed nature's law.
5. In order to get well, one must rest.
6. Today's high tension demands too much for our body to stay healthy.

7. Absolute quiet, natural foods, sleep, rest, clean fresh air, sunshine, natural water, controlled exercises and playful recreation are an absolute necessity for regaining health.
8. Don't just treat the ailment; build a perfect, healthy body.
9. To serve properly, a person must be balanced, physically, mentally and spiritually.
10. Wherever there is a disease, there is a cure right beside it.

Your home should be beautiful, for beauty heals. Unclutter, bring sunshine in, have flowers and plants. We need greenery. Do not have too much red, as it ends up making people irritable. Live surrounded by green growth, as greens are very rejuvenating. You need to have beauty around you. Be grateful and thankful, and always return blessings to life.

Blessings change our consciousness and enable us to meet our challenges more gracefully.

> "It shouldn't be the consumer's responsibility to figure out what's cruel and what's kind, what's environmentally destructive and what's sustainable. Cruel and destructive food products should be illegal. We don't need the option of buying children's toys made with lead paint, or aerosols with chlorofluorocarbons, or medicines with unlabeled side effects. And we don't need the option of buying factory-farmed animals."
>
> —Jonathan Safran Foer, Eating Animals

Spirituality and Veganism

Spiritual Growth

I truly believe that we are here to serve. It doesn't matter how we serve; the main thing is that we give of ourselves. You give to people as you learn how to give. We are here to uplift people. We have to share our knowledge with people, whether it is how to drill a waterhole in Africa or teach people how to live a healthy life. Saint Mary MacKillop said, "Never see a need without doing something about it."

Even the simplest man can offer his time as a volunteer at a soup kitchen, and therefore he becomes the most important person to the people who need volunteers. My knowledge is in nutrition, and I *know* for a fact that we don't need to eat meat in order to be healthy.

To be healthy, we need a balance of good nutritional food, peace of mind, and a positive outlook on life. In order to have peace of mind, we have to be kind and not have false ideals. In order to have a positive outlook, we must change ourselves, be willing to grow, learn to listen to other positive people and strive for a higher level of consciousness. This process will lead you automatically to better nutritional food. Your eating habits will definitely change when you change.

> *"All personal breakthroughs begin with a change in beliefs."*
> —*Anthony Robbins*

You have chosen this physical life at this time. This is just one life in many lives, and we all have many to go. Some of you might feel you've had lifetimes within this life because of who you are now, which does not resemble the person who you were years ago. Try to remember this when you become involved in "dramas" you have created yourself: grief and pain hold you stuck in your life situations. Dis-easement is a body showing that there is a dis-easement of the heart. You are on the wrong track, and you must acknowledge it. You have made the choice to be born; therefore you must take responsibility for your situation in life. You must also look at the judgement you have on yourself and others. Acknowledge the judgement. This is divine attribute, and it is the way to heal. Pain is energy. Pain is locked in the solar plexus chakra. When you judge, the energy is contained in this chakra, and you must surrender and acknowledge it and then let go, so that the pain can go out of your belly. When this process happens, it frees you up, and it allows us to be one with our godlike self.

> *"Many people are so poor that the only thing they have is money. Cultivate your spiritual growth."*
> —*Rodolfo Costa*

Meditation

For some people, this is a must, and these people meditate religiously. Other people find it very difficult and lose interest because they fall asleep. Here is a simple way to meditate if you find it difficult. There are three steps to basic meditation. You sit comfortably in a chair or on the ground. You do not have to have your legs crossed, but you must be able to sit up straight. Lean a little to the left, and then lean a little to the right. Find the position which is exactly between these two points. Then lean forward and then lean backward, and then also find the central position between these two points. Now that you are in a perfect sitting position, the aim is to have the seven chakras lined up. This means that you might have to roll your bottom in a bit and lengthen your neck. Also lengthen your spine all the way through your neck. This is the "perfect balance" position. This is a fun exercise, and you'll get to know this position really well. The idea is to relax your breathing but breathe more with intent. Pretend your body is a jug, which we are going to fill with breath, and so the stomach gets filled up first. Then the breath slowly fills up to the chest area. A good way to do this is to count to four into the abdominal area, two counts into the ribcage and two counts into the chest. Hold your breath as long as it is comfortable, relax your tongue, and then exhale slowly for the count of six from the chest and ribcage and then two from the abdomen.

Practice this, as you want this to become familiar, so you don't have to count anymore. The aim is that your energy will start flowing naturally. The second step is to pretend that there is a straight beam exactly in your middle point from your bottom chakra to the top of your head, and this beam goes perfectly through all your seven chakras. You will achieve this by sitting in the perfect balance position. Now, imagine a light coming through this beam from the bottom to the top. This might take a few sessions, because the beam might have blockages at the various chakras. Once you are able to imagine the light going right through, make this light as bright and strong as you can. Pretend that there is a window on top of your head, and you open that window and let this bright light flow out of it all over you on the outside.

"Meditation practice is like piano scales, basketball drills, ballroom dance class. Practice requires discipline; it can be tedious; it is necessary. After you have practiced enough, you become more skilled at the art form itself. You do not practice to become a great scale player or drill champion. You practice to become a musician or athlete. Likewise, one does not practice meditation to become a great meditator. We meditate to wake up and live, to become skilled at the art of living."

— Elizabeth Lesser

Once the light gets onto the floor where you are sitting, then imagine this light going back up into you through the first chakra, and so this flow of light continues going up and spilling all over you.

This is a great way to start to learn to meditate, because this still allows us to think and imagine while doing nothing. Just sitting for ten to fifteen minutes is an art in itself. What is so good about this exercise is that when you are feeling low or a bit sick, this is a great pick-me-up, because this light is actually a healing light, given freely to you from the universe. This light is full of love the universe has for you, and the more you do this exercise, the more you'll feel this love and know that we never have to struggle in life again. This light also has all of the answers, which will come to us in meditation once we learn to clear our minds.

The third stage is to allow this healing golden-white light to come from the heavens, and let it into your window on top of your head. Let this mix with your white light, which is still flowing from your bottom chakra to your top chakra on top of your head, flowing out of your window. Once you've mastered this visualization, you are ready to empty your mind and be still. Just allow things to happen. If your mind starts to wander, just bring its focus back to stillness, because it is in stillness that we can receive lessons.

Meditation deepens our self-knowledge, makes us more aware and deepens our love for and in life. When we meditate, we have more resistance to stress, lower incidence of illness, higher levels of relaxation and feelings of well-being. We sleep and digest food better. Meditation is a spiritual practice which contributes to a level of physical healing as well. Here is a short exercise which is also very beneficial: sit comfortably, close your eyes and breathe in deeply, and as you breathe out, consciously say softly, and with love in your heart: "Bless this moment." and "All is well in my life." Do this three times. Have your right hand on your heart and your left hand on your tummy as you do this. Feel your heart rate lowering, and acknowledge that this little exercise relaxed your stomach. It gives you the feeling that all is well in your world.

"Praying is talking to God, while meditating is listening to God."

—*Diana Robinson*

When a person becomes more spiritually aware, he or she inevitably experiences many awakenings. These awakenings affect every area of a person's life. It will make you think of what your intensions are with your own life. Your vision has changed. If you feel whole, then you will view the world around you differently. You'll want to contribute, and it doesn't matter how, but you feel you want to make this world a better place. Spiritual growth is all about healing—healing your own family and community but also healing yourself. You will feel connections with Mother Earth, and maybe you'll become passionate about the environment. One interesting observation: a spiritually aware person is aware of other spiritually aware people. Look at the people around you. Are they in good relationships? Do they live the right way? Who around you is peaceful? Who is environmentally friendly and who is spiritually advanced? Who lives completely? It makes you think about your own life so much more deeply. You feel more deeply in all areas.

This is where veganism comes into it, because only in veganism do we try hard not to cause suffering. If you ask yourself, "Am I a killer?", of course you are going to say no. But if you are truly honest with yourself and you ask, "Do my eating habits cause animal beings suffering?", then what would the answer be? And really, if you eat animal beings, then you are responsible for their death indirectly. The only way not to be a murderer is by not ending a life, and the only way to do that is to not eat animals. True vegans even refuse to prepare a meal for someone else that involves killing an animal being. One last question. Ask yourself, "How would it feel if you no longer contributed to the slaughter of life?" Does it feel light and full of love? Does it somehow feel like you are on a higher path?

If, by any chance, you feel justified in eating the flesh of another because you don't care or you love meat so much, then it is because you do not love yourself enough to eat food of a higher vibration.

"Life is a gift, and should be cherished, lived and experienced. Though experience often reveals itself as pain in this world, it is still purposeful, it still has its place in the evolution of our spirit."

—Michael Poeltl

Why Vegetarians Go Back to Eating Meat

Some of you have been vegans or vegetarians, and have gone back to eating meat. Usually it is because you felt like your body needed it. Let me explain this process. It is not that you crave meat and therefore you need meat; it is that a year to eighteen months prior to you eating meat again, something happened in your life that lowered your spiritual immunity, and therefore your vibrational energy changed to the same level as meat-eaters. I can even tell you what happened. You were extremely angry. Life challenged you to such a degree that it made you very angry. When this occurred, detachment of your higher self happened, and spiritual immunity was lost.

Why do we go back on the smokes? It is not that our body "needs" it. It is because a stressful situation occurred which lowered your spiritual immunity, and therefore you picked up the smokes again. This goes for anything that is bad for us. A situation occurs in our lives which makes our spiritual immunity waver. Now, if we "own" this level, then we will be strong enough not to give in, but if the time is not right yet, then we fall back to our addictions or cravings. When we want to improve our lives by giving up something, then we are actually raising our standards. Just making this decision will give us growth, and then you will be tested to see if you can stick to it or not.

The following are some of the earthbound energies that you might have experienced in the past but that are no longer a part of your life anymore: smoking, alcoholism and destructive drinking, illegal drug use, being in toxic relationships, lying, obesity, feeling victimised, gambling, laziness, gossiping, jealousy and any lifestyle choices and addictions that you know are not good for you. Some of these might be familiar to you, but all of these are destructive energies. Some people go as far as saying they "need" to smoke and call cigarettes their "little friends." Can you see that our physical body doesn't need any of these earthbound energies, *but* the body will always follow the mind. Read the last sentence again. The body will always follow the mind!

> "A man can live and be healthy without killing animals for food; therefore, if he eats meat, he participates in taking animal life merely for the sake of his appetite. And to act so is immoral."
>
> —Leo Tolstoy

We are the king of the beasts but we're a beast nevertheless. A long time ago, I was told, "If you want to do God's job, then save an animal." It was not till much later that I clicked and had my "aha" moment in regards to this saying. Yes, we are king of the beasts, but it is our job as the head of all beasts to take care of all animals in our kingdom and not to eat them. The closer our vibration is to God, the more we understand that we need to protect and help animals around us. The more we are detached from our godhead, the more separated we are from the kingdom and therefore have no problem eating animal beings instead of protecting them.

Raise your standards internally, and veganism will naturally follow. Feel the love inside of you, and recognize the higher vibration. Believe it or not, going from eating meat back to veganism also takes about a year. As you transition, don't be hard on yourself; enjoy the journey. Just be aware to be in the present.

There are many levels of energy vibrations, but once you "own" the vibration of veganism, it is hard to waver from that. If you get angry at this level, it does not lower your spiritual immunity, because anger isn't part of life anymore. Your gutter-self does not get a chance to rise, because you will get over a situation quickly and then let it go before there is an energy change. At this level, you communicate your point across rather than fight.

If you want enlightenment, if you seek a closer relationship with your higher self, you need to clean yourself internally first. This is because the mind is the last thing that gets cleaned, and therefore, in order for any "aha" moments to occur, you must detoxify. Pretend there is an invisible spiritual bar. Underneath it, you find earthbound thoughts and behaviours. Above the bar stimulates clean thinking and living. Most of us have some thought patterns and behaviours that are on both sides of the bar; it is just a question of which one you feed that will grow.

A Cherokee Legend

An old Cherokee is teaching his grandson about life. "A fight is going on inside me," he said to the boy. "It is a terrible fight and it is between two wolves. One is evil—he is anger, envy, sorrow, regret, greed, arrogance, self-pity, guilt, resentment, inferiority, lies, false pride, superiority, and ego." He continued, "The other is good—he is joy, peace, love, hope, serenity, humility, kindness, benevolence, empathy, generosity, truth, compassion, and faith. The same fight is going on inside you - and inside every other person, too."

The grandson thought about it for a minute and then asked his grandfather, "Which wolf will win?"

The old Cherokee simply replied, "The one you feed."

—Oral history mythology

Ego

Why do we hang on behaviours and practice any lifestyle below the bar? Many people are comfortable staying within their belief systems, never stepping outside their assumptions and never questioning their beliefs. We always attract situations and people into our lives that give us the opportunity to learn from an experience. It takes bravery and love for us to bring positive expansion into our lives, and that is why there is often a conflict, because behaviours below the bar are addictive.

What are addictions? Addictions are a separation from God. Addiction is an absence of love. We are addicted to the substance that gives us nurturing. When we don't love ourselves enough, we usually are unaware of the emptiness inside of us. If you are a person who needs comfort foods, works your butt off in order to keep up with the Joneses rather than work for pleasure or self-gain, has habits that shut down your senses, or needs to always keep busy, then you need to find another way to fill up that empty space within you.

One thing that often stands in the way of our wanting to change our pattern is ego. Ego is a very low energy, and it will make sure that the "I" will stay happy. The ego has very few boundaries, and its only job is to keep the "I" happy and not challenged. If the moment has gone when the "I" was happy, then the ego will find its next "happy fix," because the "I" does not like feeling empty. Escapism is a big part of the ego. The ego will protect what is most important to it, and that is false happiness. The ego will not let you be still.

Then a situation happens that makes you still, like the death of a loved one or the loss of a job or relationship. We can take the "why me?" attitude, or we can take the "why not me?" attitude and learn from the situation. We need to dig deep within ourselves and reflect on what this means for us. An unhappy situation is always forced upon us. It is a chance for us to let go of the ego and find gratitude in the things we have in our lives. It is a way we find love within ourselves and accept ourselves for who we are. We then can recognise our struggles, become humble and forgiving, be soft and wholeheartedly embrace the beautiful person we are.

> *"If you want to reach a state of bliss, then go beyond your ego and the internal dialogue. Make a decision to relinquish the need to control, the need to be approved, and the need to judge. Those are the three things the ego is doing all the time. It's very important to be aware of them every time they come up."*
>
> *—Deepak Chopra*

Every feeling we create echoes similar feelings from those around us, which can either be harmonious or not. Do not be with someone who is disharmonious; you would be better off alone. Happiness lies within us, but if we don't give ourselves time with our self, then love and self- growth cannot occur. As long as we allow the ego to distract us from going within, we are not confronted with the feelings that we have to deal with, like emptiness, loneliness, unhappiness, unhealthiness and unfulfilment.

How hard is it for you to stand naked in front of a mirror and truly love the person you see? Can you say, "I love you, respect you and admire you"? When was the last time you did something nice for this person in the mirror? I am not talking about buying a fast-food chicken dinner so you don't have to cook. I am also not talking about having a drink with your mates or buying a new pair of shoes. I am talking about meditation, yoga, making yourself a healthy juice (carrots, beetroot, celery, kale and parsley). Go for a walk in nature, sit on the beach, read a book, feel grateful, have a bath, look at a family photo album and reflect on happy times. Be by yourself, become your own best friend. Get to know yourself; it is all right to love yourself. Our old beliefs will not stand the test of time.

"You never really learn much from hearing yourself speak."
—George Clooney

No one ever develops a deeper understanding and comes into a relationship with their higher self without touching the lives of others and becoming a force of good. Deep inside of you is happiness. It is hard to find it within you, but it is impossible to find it anywhere else. Work on it; it will not let you down.

True happiness is all about showing yourself the unconditional kindness you can achieve within yourself, whereas false happiness is about showing the outside world what you can achieve outside yourself.

"We ought to do good to others as simply as a horse runs, or a bee makes honey, or a vine bears grapes season after season without thinking of the grapes it has borne."
—Marcus Aurelius

Breaking the Habit

What do you do if nothing bad ever happens in your life in order to give you the opportunity for you to grow? I call this "replacement therapy." If you want to break the habits below the bar, then replace the habit with something less destructive. If you want to become healthier, replace meat with tofu or tempeh. Replace sweets with "raw-food sweets." It is incredible how lovely this food is. Educate yourself on this subject. If you drink too much coffee and tea, replace this with rooibos and dandelion. If you feel your alcohol-drinking habits are destructive, go to AA and clean out your system with fresh vegetable juices. Try not drinking for a while; see how that is. You'll find out soon enough if there is a real problem there. Stop rewarding yourself with alcohol or cigarettes. There are so many wonderful replacement products on the market to help you stop smoking. Think about the reason you started your destructive behaviour all those years ago. Are those reasons still valid? Destructive behaviour and addictions will come knocking on your door from time to time. Remember that this is just a quick fix, and try to listen to that little voice inside, which will tell you that your behaviour will have ramifications. At the very least, it will give you a guilty feeling afterwards.

You might not even be aware of this little voice yet, so learn to listen to it, as this voice is the connection with your higher self, given to you for free from the day you were born. Your inner voice will stay with you for the rest of your life. Learn to tap into it whenever you want. Stay connected to your inner voice. Addiction is a disconnection from God, love and your higher self.

To be true to your inner self is a spiritual act, and the most spiritual thing you can do is to be the most you can be. There will be a time where you feel compelled to go within and stand alone from the group and become your "self," even if others don't like it.

Life will present you with challenges for your own growth. What you do with these opportunities is your choice, but change is natural and a necessary process. Learn to recognise patterns in your life. This is an opportunity for transformation.

Even though it is your choice which path to take, the lesson will not give you a choice, the lesson will remain the same always.

How often do we have to hear the lesson before we really hear the lesson?

—Sandra Kimler

How This Relates to Veganism—Buddha said there are four different kinds of people: those who live in the dark, those who live in the dark and are moving towards the light, those who live in the light and move towards the dark and those who live in the light.

Which one are you? If you need to make a decision, then this can be a wonderful guide.

Hopefully, this Buddhist saying will give you a clear vision and will enable you to create a new you. It can relate to physical change, mental attitude or a change in relationships. Our new thinking patterns will create new experiences. We'll create a new confidence, and our role in life changes. Be true to yourself. Show up in your life as yourself. It's okay to say no. "No" is a complete sentence. This can be very hard when it includes family. As children, we want to please our parents. We learn role-playing as we become the person our parents want us to be. Our reward is their approval. Then we grow up, and we marry a person while we are in that role, and we choose relevant jobs while in that role. We identify ourselves with the role that we are now stuck in. We become someone's wife, mother, employee, crutch. We learn how to play these roles perfectly in order to be liked or loved, and that becomes our reward.

When you want to find out who you are, then you need to peel back the layers. You most likely will find a person who is nice enough and loving enough to be her/himself. Work hard at being who you are, not on what people want you to be. Reclaim yourself, and speak your truth. You will never improve your life if you don't allow wisdom to promote you!

Wisdom is gained when you are present and aware. Then you apply common sense to day-to-day decisions. If you live in a family that is sick and overweight, then common sense should tell you that this lifestyle will not work for you in the long run. So you come to the conclusion that consuming anything that is no good for you is toxic. This can be hard for parents to hear. It is an insult to your mother, who has always given you the best she could.

> *"I think 'vegan' is a beautiful word. It is more than just a descriptor for our diet. I see it as a visible template for an ethical, healthy, responsible, and rational life. Because it describes our character. It says we do not take the life of another living being to satisfy our wants."*
>
> *—Phillip Wollen*

Eating is both a physical and a spiritual act. Our food should nourish both body and soul. As babies, our first nourishing experience is in the arms of our mothers. We not only partake in food, we also partake in relationship strengthening. As we grow up, this relationship continues with the family, but now we sit around the table for dinner. I think it is a real shame that so many families sit in front of the TV while eating dinner. When we do eat with the family around the table, the connection is more about sharing stories as well as food. It is usually a positive experience.

Right across the world, celebrations always involve food and gathering together. This enhances our understanding of each other, our community, our family and our culture. Because meat has always been a big part of family gatherings, it is often family who will feel threatened the most when you are changing. Our parents will tell us meat has always been part of tradition. Their story has become their truth. We all have our own family rituals, and the intention is to keep family traditions alive. However, it is your job to make yourself happy, and you cannot let your peers decide what you eat or do not eat, regardless of tradition. Not many people have the will to change, and we often don't change because we were brought up on meats and dairy products, and therefore, that's the way it is. Dependence on the past supports systems already in place.

Our forefathers ate meat, and our children will grow up on it. Well, that is a lousy excuse. I am Dutch, and there are no bigger meat-eating, milk-drinking fools than they. Well, most of the Western world, really. And look at them—they are sick with cold and flu, or they are having a knee replacement. They have arthritis or are depressed. Most of them are overweight, with hormone and thyroid imbalances, and lots of them have had cancer. The doctor happily gives a pill for everything. People are not getting better; our society is getting sicker and sicker. Is no one putting one and one together? Maybe it is the food we are eating.

So what if our fathers ate meat? Back then, they also didn't eat all the other junk that we eat today. Maybe their bodies could cope with the acidity of animal protein. Meals were a lot simpler, there was less stress and digestion was better.

> *"Look into the depths of your own soul and learn first to know yourself, then you will understand why this illness was bound to come upon you and perhaps you will thenceforth avoid falling ill."*
>
> —Sigmund Freud

The next thing is that you decide you are going to be eating healthier. Once you set yourself up to change, you'll find out how much there is to learn. Fourteen million Australians are overweight. Our kids will have a shorter life expectancy than us. Not only that, these figures are expected to rise. By 2025, 80 percent of Australians will be overweight. It is costing Australia billions, and all we have to do to make it better is stop eating animal protein. Even if we eat less animal protein, it would be better. There is Meatfree Mondays Australia, which was launched in Australia in 2009. We are the eighth country to be running this campaign. Take a look at: meatfreeweek.org

If each American would participate in Meatless Mondays, it would save 1.4 billion animal beings every year. It's a start, and even this small change will bring awareness. It is a small change, but it will bring healthier eating habits and with it, enlightenment.

> *"You may believe that you are responsible for what you do, but not for what you think. The truth is that you are responsible for what you think, because it is only at this level that you can exercise choice. What you do comes from what you think."*
>
> —A Course in Miracles

When we become mindful of the food we eat, we find that all aspects in our lives will transform with spiritual intention. Use the "replacement theory" here. Replace chicken with tofu; replace animal stock with vegetable stock; replace meat sausages with vegan sausages; replace bacon bits in our salad with sunflower kernels. Instead of ham-and-cheese sandwiches, have tomato and avocado, and replace beef stir-fry with tempeh stir-fry. Update your thinking, and stay open to new experiences. A vegan diet results in significantly less heart disease, cancer, diabetes, kidney disease, immune disorders and osteoporosis. To become vegan might seem overwhelming. Kathy Freston says that we need to "lean" into veganism. See yourself as a changing vehicle. Let the new become the old; let go and embrace the next stage. See yourself as forever improving physically and spiritually. Make the decision not to acknowledge old habits anymore. Shut the door on them, and breathe in the new. Make a commitment to say no to foods and drinks that don't benefit your health. Find an environment that encourages health.

> *"You'll never find the right path in life if you don't let go of the wrong one."*
>
> *—Anonymous*

Food Vibrations

Everything has its own signature vibration. The vibration between meat and vegan food is very different. High-vibrational foods include fresh organic fruit and veggies, nuts and seeds, berries and alkaline foods. Lowest-vibrational foods are any animal-protein foods. Meat is the densest, lowest-energy of all, because it is extremely acidic. Other low-energy foods are all cooked, baked, boiled and barbecued foods.

You can also measure light in cells. This is called biophoton energy. Dr. Fritz Albert Popp, a German scientist, found that biophotons in healthy people were significantly stronger than in unhealthy people.

In *Creating Peace by Being Peace,* Gabriel Cousens cites the biophoton readings of people on sharply varying diets. While a person eating a diet of junk food only had a reading of roughly one thousand units of biophotonic radiation, the average reading from a person eating live or raw wild foods was about eighty-three thousand units. He also discovered that cooked or irradiated food emitted virtually no biophotons.

Popp found that organic foods growing in the wild emitted twice as many biophotons as cultivated organic crops, while the latter gave off five times as much biophotonic energy as commercially grown foods. The average baby had forty-three thousand, which was the same as a person who ate a good plant-based diet.

One person who ate high-vibrational foods and wild herbs and fasted regularly had 114,000 biophoton energy. What do you think happens to a person who eats a lot of "low-energy foods"? They are your average first-world adults, going to doctors, complaining and depressed. How simple is it to be vibrant?

> *"We can make a commitment to promote vegetables and fruits and whole grains on every part of every menu. We can make portion sizes smaller and emphasize quality over quantity. And we can help create a culture—imagine this—where our kids ask for healthy options instead of resisting them."*
> —*Michelle Obama*

So how is veganism related to spirituality? You can be spiritual and still eat animal beings, but you'll stay stagnant at that level. You stay stagnant because eating meat and bringing suffering has karma attached to it. And what is karma? It is the life lessons that keep coming back to us until we learn from it. Karma happens below the bar. Above the bar is just growth. Spiritual veganism evolved because people could not hurt animal beings, directly or indirectly. Every animal knows it is about to be slaughtered at the abattoir.

Imagine how scared the animals are. First, the animal was removed from its place of residence, often roughly and without respect or love. All animals live in families and have a strong bond. When some of them get removed, it causes panic in the group because of the separation. Once at the abattoir, there is the smell of death, blood, fear and helplessness. Each species of animal has its own cries and it echoes with the cries and bleats of those communicating danger to the others. We turn a blind eye, because people want to eat meat, but in your own opinion, what level of vibration does this have? Eleven million hens are confined in cages in Australia no bigger than themselves. They will never know what it is to stretch their legs or wings.

Meat-eaters consume this energy. Each bite of meat contains the vibration of adrenaline, a hormone produced by the body when an animal being is in stress. Each bite of meat contains the vibration of fear and misery. You as a meat-eater consume these vibrations. Are you really okay with that? Can you see enlightenment for yourself when you are a cause of this suffering? This is no different from the suffering forced upon people in slavery, child labour and gender discrimination.

It is people causing suffering to others, which is wrong, and it doesn't matter whether they are human beings or animal beings. It is wrong, and if you can't relate to that, then you lack compassion and empathy.

"I became a vegetarian after realizing that animals feel afraid, cold, hungry and unhappy like we do. I feel very deeply about vegetarianism and the animal kingdom. It was my dog Boycott who led me to question the right of humans to eat other sentient beings."

— César Chávez

The power of compassion lets us realise that animal beings are the same as us. When we show compassion, it makes us feel good. Compassion is associated with the pleasure area in the brain. Compassionate practices improve our health. James Doty, a neurosurgeon, talks about a study that was done with those over the age of sixty-five. Those who volunteered to help others were compared to those who did not. In his own words:

"Their longevity was doubled compared to the group who did not. This research gives us a hint that being kind or compassionate leads to a decrease in stress hormones, a boost in your immune system, and is associated with increased longevity. This is fascinating. Understand what compassion is, for example, in your family. Who do you love the most, and whose welfare are you most interested in? And then expanding the circle further and further out to the end, it encompasses essentially all humans and sentient beings. It does take continued effort. But think about when you yourself have done an act like that to somebody, and you see on their face how they've responded.

When you care for somebody in an authentic way, deep in your heart, it stays with you, and you can relive it. It makes you want to do it again to somebody else. I call that *transcendence;* it is a sense that you have a purpose in life, that the act of connecting with another defines your purpose, that we're in fact all one. When you have that sense, that is the thing that gives you happiness and joy". Compassion is being at the same level, looking them in the eye, and saying we're the same, and that defines your humanity; that is true compassion.

We know that an individual has this incredible sense of connection to people, but only within his or her in-group. So the key is, how do you expand that in-group to a larger circle? That's an area of interest for Dave DeSteno at Northeastern University in the United States. His research shows that if you can look for things in common with people outside of your in-group, you'll likely find multiple things, and this exercise decreases our feelings of separateness. Each time you do that, it actually decreases the sense of separateness.

We arc all one. When you have the ability to see separateness, or when you give a being (human or animal) the sense that the other has lesser value, *what does that say about you?* Please learn to keep an open heart to all beings.

Compassion is the start of all spiritual work, because our consciousness feels joy, which then increases the desire to practice more goodness.

My wish is for people to do the right thing, to live the right life, to be good people for goodness' sake. It takes courage for us to be good people. It is not our beliefs that make us good people; it is our actions that make us good. We must trust in our highest good.

My wish is for you to ingest only food that preserves peace and well-being inside your body. A vegan diet transforms an individual, both physically and spiritually, and this has many positive affects in society. A vegan diet is an alkaline diet, but to be a good vegan, you must bring philosophy and a peaceful lifestyle together and live in harmony.

> *"In fact, if one person is unkind to an animal it is considered to be cruelty, but where a lot of people are unkind to animals, especially in the name of commerce, the cruelty is condoned and, once large sums of money are at stake, will be defended to the last by otherwise intelligent people."*
> —Ruth Harrison, Animal Machines

Environment and Veganism

Unsustainability

I do not have to tell you that our Earth is overpolluted and overpopulated. We've passed the tipping point for biodiversity loss. Our oceans are dying, our ice is melting and our virgin forests are lost forever.

Every day, for all 7 billion of us, we leave an environmental and an ecological footprint. If the 7 billion of us would try harder to minimise this footprint, then the Earth could heal, even if it is ever so slightly. Environmental toxicity makes us sick. It lowers our immunity. The statistics are horrifying, and I encourage you to look at these statistics on the internet for yourself, because a whole world of human-caused destruction will open up to you. Take your pick; we've ruined everything we could ruin, to a certain extent. What I find even more disturbing is that we spend hundreds of billions of dollars on finding answers to preserving what little natural environment we have left. Why not spend money educating people about where in their lives they are polluting the most. Why not educate people on the everyday habits they have which cause pollution and what they can do to minimise the global environmental burden. Most people would be open to living a life of environmentally supportive behaviour with environmentally supportive values. So why aren't we?

The reason why we are so slow to change is simple: we don't like change, and therefore, we see in life the things that support our belief system. The government surely won't educate people, because it would mean financial losses (or so they think). We need to educate ourselves, be responsible for what we do and eat. Our Earth is fragile, and we are using its resources at a rate that is unsustainable. We clear land all over the world, to have animals graze on it for us to eat at a later stage. It sickened me when I saw a documentary on the huge amount of the Amazon's virgin jungle that was removed to make room for export beef to graze on. Other parts of the Amazon were logged to grow soybeans and grains to feed these animals, while there were people starving on the same continent. The wealthy farmers from Germany who owned the land did with it whatever they wanted. When they were asked whether they felt bad about what they were doing, they said they didn't and that those who wanted to preserve the jungle should buy it for themselves.

> *"In a few decades, the relationship between the environment, resources and conflict may seem almost as obvious as the connection we see today between human rights, democracy and peace."*
>
> *—Wangari Maathai (1940–2011),*
> *environmental activist, first African woman*
> *to receive the Nobel Peace Prize in 2004*

In Australia, the situation isn't any better. Almost 60 percent of the continent is used for grazing animals which are going to be used for meat. We are continuing to clear forests and bushland for this purpose. This results in a huge amount of what is already a fragile habitat loss. Erosion is a major problem, and according to the CSIRO, a massive 92 percent of all land degradation in Australia is caused by animal industries.

Australia is such a dry continent, with regular droughts and water restrictions all the time. Did you know that it took 5,500 litres of water to produce a single kilogram of beef? It takes 5,000 litres of water to produce 1 kilo of cheese, 3,900 litres of water to produce 1 kilo of chicken, and 6,000 litres of water to produce a kilogram of pork. For one glass of milk, it takes four thousand of the same glasses of water to produce it. To produce 1 kilo of potatoes, it takes 630 litres of water; 1 kilo of corn takes 650 litres of water; and a kilo of apples takes 70 litres of water. On average, 1 kilogram of veggies uses 322 litres of water to be produced. [4]]

Animal products have a larger water footprint than crop products. The same is true when we look at the water footprint per calorie. The average water footprint per calorie for beef is twenty times larger than for cereals and starchy roots. You get the picture; a vegan diet requires a quarter of the water compared to that of a meat-eater.

Not long ago there was a large movement away from eating steak to eating fish and seafood. This led to overfishing. Modern technology provided a way we could fish more intensely. Unfortunately, the techniques also destroyed the ocean environment by using dredges, long lines, purse seine nets, trawl nets and gillnets. The problem with this is that there is an enormous amount of "by-catch." Many species are now facing extinction due to being a by-catch. By-catch is not the targeted fish species and includes turtles, dolphins, seals, sea birds, whales, dugongs and sharks. An estimated ninety-seven thousand tonnes of these non-targeted animals are caught in Australian waters alone every year. That is just in Australian waters. The bottom-trawling devastates the ocean floor, destroying everything in its path and eliminates hiding, feeding and breeding areas for so many sea species. This is a global environmental problem. All this by-catch was potential food for other sea species. What we've seen across the globe is that there is not enough food left for seals, penguins, bears, and big and small fish to eat. Species are dying because of it, or they are smaller and weaker than their parents. [5]

"The human voice can never reach the distance that is covered by the still small voice of conscience."

—*Mahatma Gandhi*

What we've also seen across the globe is the difference in the catch caught by fishermen from small fishing villages. The sad thing is that this is their livelihood, and they have been fishermen for generations. These villages rely 100 percent on the catch that comes in every day. There has been such a decline that the people from these villages are struggling to stay alive. A lot of fishing villages have disappeared. Fishermen now have to go out further, where the waters are far more dangerous, to catch a little bit of fish.

Some people started to eat fish from fish farms, thinking this is a better option. These farmed fish eat wild fish, and for every kilogram of farmed fish, it takes five kilograms of wild fish to produce it. Apart from that, captive fish swim in small captive areas. This results in faecal contamination, promoting diseases and the spread of parasites.

Scientists Ransom Myers and Boris Worm have reported that 90 percent of all large fish in our oceans are now gone.

According to the UNFAO, governments around the world heavily subsidize their fishing industries to the tune of US $29 billion that's 29,000,000,000 dollars. One in four Australians takes fish-oil supplements. The sad thing is that the omega 3 isn't effective at all and is an unjustifiable expense to your health and the environment. Plant-based omega 3 will benefit you more and will give you optimal health. Walnuts, flaxseed, canola oil, soybeans and lots of other plants like lettuce, broccoli, kale, spinach and legumes like mung, kidney, navy, pinto, lima beans, peas and split peas have it. Also, citrus fruits, melons and cherries contain not only omega 3 but also omega 6 and omega 9. When you have these three omegas in the right ratios, it is effective against cardiac problems. But Western diet overloads on omega 6, and this results in arthritic pain, cardiovascular disease, type-2 diabetes, obesity, irritable bowel syndrome and inflammatory bowel disease, rheumatoid arthritis, asthma, cancer, psychiatric disorders and many more inflammatory diseases. Fish oil is also very acidic, and this is why it causes inflammation. Also, animal-derived omega 3 causes bleeding and bruising. So fish oil is actually harmful for you.

"Fish can be contaminated with various toxins including metals like mercury and lead, industrial chemicals like PCBs, and even pesticides like DDT and dieldrin. Some fish are so contaminated that the federal government and environmental protection agencies recommend limited or no consumption of fish. As an example, wild-caught Alaskan salmon is a relatively safe fish to eat, whereas farmed Atlantic salmon is one of the worst."

—Tracy Shields

The new craze is krill oil. This little crustacean lives in the icy waters around the Antarctic. It is considered to be better than fish oil, because the absorption rate is better. Did you know that it is what a krill eats that gives us the benefit? Krill eats grasses of the sea. Yes, the bit that is good for us are the greens that krill eats. Doesn't it make more sense for us just to eat our greens in order to be healthy and not disturb what is the last pristine waters and create heat where we really don't want it? Krill is also the main food for whales, penguins, fish, squid and seals. Krill weigh 2 grams, and every year we remove 150,000 to 200,000 tonnes of krill, and this too produces enormous amounts of by-catch.

Wouldn't you know it—nature's vegan food gives us the perfect way to be healthy. That is probably why there is so little heart disease when people follow a vegan diet.

"How wonderful it is that nobody needs to wait a single moment before starting to improve the world."

—Anne Frank

Did you know that one-third of the world's population is starving, one-third is fed and one-third is overfed? Did you know that one-third of the world's edible grain harvest is fed to the livestock industry? What if we took beef out of the picture? Then we could give that one-third of edible grain to the one-third of starving people.

We turn a blind eye to this little statistic, because the first world loves to eat meat. Twenty-five thousand children die every day from starvation.

Nearly 70 billion animals are slaughtered every year. (This does not include sea animals.) These animals need to eat, but they also need to drink. At 93 percent of the total global water consumption, the largest sector using our fresh water is agriculture, with nearly 50 percent of all water use being taken up by livestock. Half of all the water used on Earth is given to the animals raised and then killed for us to eat. How much do we use for our own drinking purposes? Less than 1 percent of all water consumed annually. What if we took beef out of the picture? Then we could give that 50 percent of fresh water to those who don't have it.

We turn a blind eye to this little statistic, because the first world loves to eat meat. Forty-five hundred children die each day from unsafe, dirty water.

Every time we buy meat, or any other animal product for that matter, it is a "yes" vote to keep that industry going. It is a "yes" vote to keep destroying the environment; it is a "yes" vote to keep you unhealthy.

Governments are trying to make us aware of the impact we have on the environment by telling us to recycle, reuse, take shorter showers, change to efficient light-globes, use solar, drive environmentally better cars, turn heating down, Look for higher "A" ratings on fridges, freezers, washing machines and donate to companies that offer carbon-footprint offset credits. But the governments fail to address the one thing that is the most unsustainable of all: *what we eat!*

So what can you do? According to the documentary "Meat the Truth," if all Australians reduced meat intake by *one* day per week, the savings in greenhouse-gas emissions would be equivalent to the greenhouse gases emitted from 7 million plane trips between Brisbane and Perth!

If all Australians reduced meat intake by *two* days per week, the savings in greenhouse-gas emissions would be equivalent to replacing every single household appliance (fridges, freezers, microwaves, dishwashers, dryers, washing machines, etc.) with energy-efficient ones.

If all Australians reduced meat intake by *three* days per week, the savings in greenhouse-gas emissions would be equivalent to saving 21 megatonnes of greenhouse-gas emissions, which is more than would be saved if every single car was replaced with a Prius.

If all Australians reduced meat intake by *four* days per week, the savings in greenhouse-gas emissions would be equivalent to halving the nationwide domestic use of electricity, gas, oil, petroleum and kerosene combined.

If all Australians reduced meat intake by *five* days per week, the savings in greenhouse-gas emissions would be equivalent to planting 1 billion trees in your backyard and allowing them to grow for ten years.

If all Australians reduced meat intake by *six* days per week, the savings in greenhouse-gas emissions would be equivalent to: saving the total electricity use of every Australian household combined.

If all Australians reduced meat intake by *seven* days per week, the savings in greenhouse-gas emissions would be equivalent to: taking every single car off the road.

Meat-eating is nothing more than an ego-based practice.

"An organic vegan diet produces 94% less greenhouse gas emissions than the average meat and dairy diet."
—Foodwatch report, 2009[6]

Ethics and Veganism

Ethics and the Abattoir

Ethical systems deal with morals. This can involve physical issues (it is morally wrong to kill someone); or it can involve a mental issue (it is ethically wrong to wish bad luck onto someone). We judge our actions against what we as a society have proposed is right and what is wrong. These ethical proposals differ according to each situation. A good example is this: when a person hurts an animal, it is considered to be cruel, and our laws will punish that person, but when there is a group of people being cruel to animals in the name of big-money commerce (as in abattoirs and live-animal export), then it is condoned to be cruel to animals.

What I've come to realize is that we still have many people below the spiritual bar (page 102). In this group, there are still many young souls who are at such a low vibration that working at abattoirs is a good place for them. I am not judging here; it is just that they are attracted to this type of work. As long as there is an element of this vibration still within us, this practice will continue to be. Going undercover in an abattoir is easy, as there are a lot of people who can do this work only for a little while, and so there is a high staff turnover.

So goes the story in a pig abattoir in England. I've been told that folk who work at abattoirs are not the kind of people you want as an enemy. In this particular abattoir, pigs are killed the conventional way on one side, and on the other side of the building, cows are killed in the kosher way. Pigs are held in holding bays, and then about twenty pigs each time are led into a small area called the killing floor. This is a very dirty, smelly and bloody area, which consists of a concrete floor where the killing is done. There are two men who each carry two electric steel rods, one in either hand. The idea is that they put the rods on either side of the pig, near the front where the heart is, and electrocute the animal. The pig goes stiff straight away, doesn't feel anything beyond this point. The pig then is dragged to an area in this room where it is hung up on a chain which is like a conveyer belt, and then the pig goes out of view. I have been told they are then boiled to make the skin soft and the hair disappear, and then the butchering starts. Acceptable to some people in theory.

"When the time comes for slaughter, pigs are forced onto transport trucks that travel for many miles through all weather extremes. Many die of heat exhaustion in the summer or arrive frozen to the inside of the truck in the winter. According to industry reports, more than 1 million pigs die in transport each year, and an additional 420,000 are crippled by the time they arrive at the slaughterhouse."
—People for the Ethical Treatment of Animals (PETA)

So, these two men walk around the killing floor filled with twenty pigs or so, and they are doing their job as quickly as they can. They kill four hundred pigs per hour (more than six per minute). A typical slaughterhouse kills over a thousand pigs per hour. These two men are talking to each other, cracking jokes, laughing and mucking around. Their focus is not on the pigs or that they should kill the animal as effectively as possible. As a joke, Guy 1 watches Guy 2 as Guy 2 touches a pig to get the pig into the electrocution position. Guy 1 thinks it's funny to touch that same pig with one of his electrocution rods. A blast of electricity goes through the pig, as well as Guy 2, who crumples over in pain and swears out loud. Guy 1 thinks this was hilarious, and both men end up laughing about it as Guy 2 says, "You got me good that time."

The pig, on the other hand, knows how much these rods hurt, and even though it can't really stand up anymore, it tries to get away, squealing. It has alarmed the other pigs in the room, and they too try to escape. It is sad to watch the other pigs in the room, because they know their fate. Pigs are very smart and sensitive beings. The two men are in their own world and not concentrating on the right electrocution style at all, as one rod touches the pig's ribcage and the other rod touches the pig's face. As a result, the pig does not go stiff; it squeals out in excruciating pain. It can't stand up anymore and gets kicked a few times but also gets dragged to be chained up and taken away towards the scalding tank. This pig was very much still alive, but no one took any notice. At least 10 percent of the pigs that came to this abattoir were "downers." These are pigs that are seriously sick or injured, and they are so weak that they cannot walk or stand up. They are constantly touched by the electric prods and kicked in order to move along.

When asked about the killing of pigs, Guy 1 said openly how he felt about it, and he admitted that he liked to kill. He said that if he could not come to work every day and kill, then he would be in jail for hurting or killing someone. His job was an "outlet" for all the aggression and anger he felt inside. When he was asked about animal welfare, he shrugged his shoulders and said that he was there to do a job.

> "I seen them take those stunners—they're about as long as a yardstick—and shove it up the hog's ass… They do it with cows, too… And in their ears, their eyes, down their throat … They'll be squealing and they'll just shove it right down there."
> —Gail Eisnitz, from her book Slaughterhouse[4]

At no stage did these two men show compassion, not even to the pigs that were hurt in the transportation from the factory farm to the abattoir as they were lying in the filth of the holding pen. They were extremely stressed and were foaming from the mouth. One guy picked up a brick that looked like a bessa brick and dropped it as hard as he could on the pig's face. I think the idea was to knock the pig out, but it took four or five goes before the pig's body went limp. On a spiritual level, we still need abattoirs because there are people with the same vibrational level as what the abattoirs offer. For those who eat meat, the vibration isn't any better, because every person knows how cruel these places are. Not only that, but meat-eaters put these people in jobs. Meat-eaters are the cause of these violent careers, and abattoir workers are only there because of demand. These two men treated these beautiful, peaceful and kind pigs with cruelty beyond words. You stop eating pigs, then you stop this practice.

> "Hogs that didn't get stunned properly get up to the scalding tank, hit the water and start screaming and kicking. Sometimes they thrash so much they kick water out of the tank ... Sooner or later they drown. There's a rotating arm that pushes them under, no chance for them to get out. I'm not sure if they burn to death before they drown, but it takes them a couple of minutes to stop thrashing."
> —Gail Eisnitz, from her book Slaughterhouse[7]

What was most disturbing was the behaviour of the organic pigs that came off the truck from the farm. There was a distinct difference between these and the conventionally raised pigs, as the organic pigs were used to being in a more pleasant situation. These pigs had a higher sense of awareness. It was like they instinctively knew they were going to be killed, and they tried with all their might to escape. They didn't walk in lines and follow the pack. They were extremely frightened, compared to the factory-farmed pigs. One organic pig started vomiting as it was kicked to move along, and then it actually began choking on its own vomit, but the workers had no tolerance for this and hit and kicked the animal even harder. If you are a person who eats organic pig because you think it is better, let me assure you that they all go to the same slaughterhouse. I would say don't eat pig at all, because choosing between two evils is still choosing an evil. As for the factory-farmed pigs, it was the first time they saw daylight and hadn't breathed in ammonia-laden air. For them, this was a whole new experience.

They had never walked, so their leg muscles were weak, but they felt safe enough with all the other pigs in the holding bay. That was until they were brought to the killing floor.

On the other side of the abattoir building was the area where cows were killed the kosher way. This area was run by a rabbi, whom I found to be a pleasant man with a soft voice. He explained that they allow one cow in at a time, so that the other cows do not see any of the killing. He had a sharp knife, and with one very quick strike, he cut the cow's oesophagus, the trachea, carotid arteries and the jugular veins. He then wiped his knife clean, ready for the next cow. He said that he did this job not because he liked it but because of the high need for halal and kosher meat. He said that if this needs to be done, then he will do it as painlessly and quickly as possible out of respect for the animal.

He disapproved of what was happening next door, with the pig killings, and he called them clowns with no respect for an animal that was about to die. I did agree with him on that point, but this cow still suffered a great deal, as it was not stunned before the stabbing. Their religious laws state that the animal should be left alone to bleed to death, but that wasn't the case at all. The cow that had just been stabbed collapsed onto the floor, and this steel floor tilted, so the cow slid off it onto a lower area, where it was hung by one of its hind legs. This cow was fully conscious as it bled to death.

I failed to see how this was kosher or halal, as the requirements for this type of slaughter were not (not even close to it) followed correctly. Not only did they not comply with kosher or halal standards, they also did not comply with slaughterhouse standards, as it clearly states that if the animal is not stabbed correctly or it moves around too much, then it must be stunned. None of the cows that were stabbed incorrectly were stunned, and no one helped these animals to a quick death. Instead, there was a lot of blood splatter as the cows fought for their lives.

> "I've hit cows till their bones start breaking, while they were still alive. Bringing them around the corner and they get stuck up in the doorway, just pull them till their hide be ripped, till the blood just drip on the steel and concrete. Breaking their legs … And the cow be crying with its tongue stuck out. They pull him till his neck just pop.
>
> "I seen guys take broomsticks and stick it up the cow's behind, screwing them with a broom."
>
> —Gail Eisnitz, from her book Slaughterhouse[8]

Last word

Since eating is such a huge part of our lives, it is a great way for us to practice being conscious of what we put into our mouths. We eat three times a day minimum and snack all day through. Next time you eat, ask your higher self if he or she approves. Ask yourself, is this cruel-free? Was there any suffering? Was it environmentally friendly? How much carbon footprint and water print did I clock up, eating this product? There are many levels you can better yourself on, and the start of this awareness is being conscious of the fact that you want to change.

Being ethical, in its simplest form, is doing the right thing. It's making decisions that would have our higher self bestow blessings upon us. Read this sentence again, and feel the high vibration coming from it. What do you feel it would mean for you if you lived a life of doing the right thing? Don't you think your perception of your reality in this world would change? What would this mean for your children, spouse, family and friends if the intention behind every decision you made was for the greater good? What would it mean to your community, your shire, state, country, your world? What would it mean to the world if from now on, every decision you make is enlightenment-based rather than ego-based? Well, I can tell you that your world would be a better place, and everyone around you would not only benefit from your goodness but also learn from it. This has a snowball effect where you pay forward with your loving goodness. The people around you will do the same, and that is how your community will benefit. This will spread right throughout the world. This is how you make a difference and make this world a better place.

> "Veganism functioned as a purification. When you eat animals you are more under the law of necessity. You are heavy, you gravitate more towards the earth. When you are a vegan you are light and you are more under the law of grace, under the law of power, and you start gravitating towards the sky."
>
> —Osho

Part Three

We've known for more than twenty years that the immune system of a vegan is superior to that of a meat-eater. The German Cancer Research Centre found that although vegans and meat-eaters had the same amount of disease-fighting white blood cells, the immune cells of vegans were twice as effective in destroying cancer and virus-infected cells as those of meat-eaters.

In the United States alone, the annual cost of meat- and dairy-based diseases is around 1 trillion dollars and increasing every year. All animal protein is acidic, and it keeps our bodies in a constant state of inflammation. This is an ideal environment for cancer to thrive. A vegan diet is a plant-based diet, and therefore you get all the antioxidants that are critical for neutralizing acidity. Vegans get far more natural fibre, which cleans our systems perfectly.

Animals show us that they really hate slavery, captivity and a lack of freedom. Animals will weaken in captivity and in some cases will die.

In the case of our pets, we make a deal with them to compensate for their loss of freedom. We give them food, shelter, company, love and attention.

This doesn't happen to the animals we eat or use for our own gains. We give them the very minimum, just enough to keep them alive until we kill them. We give them a miserable life, and they truly feel their loss of freedom, their loss of the right to exhibit their natural behaviour.

Freedom is a powerful force, and everything we do, animal beings as well as human beings, is directed towards freedom. As humans, we often view having money as a form of freedom. With lots of money comes power and the freedom to direct money to what you feel is worthy.

I must tell you that I know very little about politics, and the following story is evidence of that. When 9/11 happened, it was the first time there was such an attack on America, and it shook the world up. In fact, the world has never been the same since. Of course, I acknowledged the fact that three thousand people died, but I must admit that I had a hint of optimism inside of me. It was the first time that the whole world stood still for a couple of days, waiting for what was going to happen next. President Bush had decisions to make, and everyone was just waiting for that. To me, this was a chance for world peace. It was a chance for America to ask why this happened and learn from this experience. What if Bush declared world peace? What if he had said, "Those responsible will be punished, but from this day onward, let's put laws into place that ensure peace, communication, forgiveness and sharing."?

But of course, he did not. Did you know that globally, governments spend $1,738,000,000,000,000 every year on military alone? This extraordinary amount of money goes into preparation in case of war every year. America alone has $600 billion to spend, and he was going to spend some of it on finding "weapons of destruction." That is little consolation to the 7.6 million children who die every year of hunger and the 925 million people who haven't enough to eat. Imagine if this world *really* was his priority. He would invest in peace, and he would invest in the development of green power. Why not then set up environmentally friendly villages for poor people, teach them how to grow their own food? On a vegetarian diet, there is more than enough room to grow food for 8 billion people. On a vegan diet, there is enough to grow for 12 billion people. Why not invest in global tree-planting, regenerate forests, invest in ocean protection, invest in climate change, teach people how to minimize their carbon footprint and water print? He could invest in teaching people how to eat environmentally friendly foods. Imagine how many jobs that would create. How wonderful to have people teach peace, teach equality, which includes the equal rights of animals and environmental places. Teach people how to re-use, recycle and practice accountability. People can become aware of global overpopulation and how this is so destructive to our Mother Earth. Laws could be put into place that this is the higher focus and is above ego, greed and religion, which are the only reasons for war.

Of course, this did not happen and won't happen in this lifetime. But nothing stops us from implementing some of these peace rules into our everyday lives today. I would love for the politicians of today to ask the question: What would the peacemakers do? What decision would the Dalai Lama make? Mother Teresa, Nelson Mandela, Jesus, Gandhi, Dr. Martin Luther King Jr., Abraham Lincoln—what would they say about all of this, and how far removed is the decision to do something differently to that of our peacemakers?

What this process allows is for us to connect with our higher selves. Connecting with our higher selves feels great. Being peaceful is what we do for ourselves and not for anyone else. Ego has no place in this level of thinking and living. Ego gives us little pleasures that don't last. The feeling we get from our higher selves is a deeper feeling of delight that stays with us. At this level, you live in a spiritual place. I don't mean you are a tree-hugging hippie now who sings "Kumbaya." (Not that there is anything wrong with it. I have the highest respect for people who are dedicated in this way.) But you then are a person with his/her feet on the ground, who is very much aware of the connection to all that is out there, and you have no place for ego. You are aware of the inner growth within yourself. Every person is obligated to understand himself. Understanding yourself means that you understand where your thoughts came from, like your upbringing or other influences. Everything we do in this world has an emotion and a thought attached to it. This is also the case with eating. When we eat, the emotion is that we like the food, it fills us up; the thought is that we are going to enjoy sitting down with family and friends and sharing a lovely meal. As we become aware, there is going to be a time when meat and dairy is *not* going to give us that lovely feeling. We will "sense the intention" behind that food, what energy comes from that food. Next time you eat meat, be really aware of how that meat came to be on your plate. After you eat this meat, how does it feel for this to be inside you? The meat you purchased is a product of misery and slavery. The food these animals ate is GM food; it weakens their system. The animal you ate was full of toxins, and when the animal was brought to its killing place, it was scared, with adrenaline flowing through the whole body.

This is what you put into your body. It was not a circumstance of beauty and peace. Which one do you feel our higher selves would prefer?

Or will you decide that maybe for now you will stick to what your physical needs are and not your spiritual needs.

> *Ego is attachment to oneself and spirituality is our inner connection to what is out there.*
>
> *—Sandra Kimler.*

No one will change if they don't want to. This is our freedom. It is our freedom to eat meat or not. What is *not* our freedom are the lessons that are placed onto our path in order for us to grow. Growth is always for the better, and we always learn from it; we become more aware from the lessons. If we do not see the lesson, then it will come on our path again and again. Therefore, I will never feel bad about promoting veganism, because I will not come onto the path of those who have absolutely no interest in this subject. When the student is ready, the teacher will appear. The road to spirituality must be in total freedom.

We have come into an age that requires us to connect to everything all at once, and veganism is part of that. For thousands of years, we have developed ourselves according to our ego, and it resulted in the state the world is in now. *Love and treat your neighbour as yourself* is a part of veganism, because it opens us up to love and connection. It shows us a way of internal consciousness on a planetary level, which we show on an external level, through our behaviour.

When we live a vegan lifestyle, we connect with the environmental forces. We also connect to ethical forces. We become healthier and therefore feel better about ourselves, and of course, we connect with all animal beings. This leads to a connected, humane world. When we are open to this, we can start to heal physically, emotionally and spiritually. Doctors will become more open to "functional" medicine. Pills just don't work. Doctors of the future must look at the whole person and understand where the disease comes from, instead of giving a pill which does take away the symptom but not the cause.

Disease can be stress-related, and in order to be healthy, one simply needs to learn to meditate. Disease can be environmentally related, such that a person must leave the city and live in clean air. Our nervous systems are all different from each other, and what heals one does not necessarily heal another. Doctors must study nutrition and stop listening to our dairy and meat suppliers, who pay enormous amounts of money. They must understand that a thyroid problem is an emotional hurt-related symptom and can be fixed up easily when the person recognizes this.

Making a person take a pill for the rest of his life is ridiculous. Doctors need to study iridology, so they can tell a patient what caused her asthma. It could be that the person's back is out of alignment, and all it needs is for a chiropractor or an osteopath to line it up again, which causes normal blood flow, which in turn takes away all mucus which caused the asthma in the first place. But instead, they prescribe an asthma inhaler or pill which has bromide in it. Please look this up on Google (The Bromide Dominance Theory) and familiarize yourself with bromide if you or your child has an asthma inhaler. The fact that doctors give us inhalers is very disturbing in itself, because they are not treating what caused it in the first place. Doctors should learn the art of "tapping," this is a practice that asks the body why it is sick; doctors should understand that we are sick because of stress, diet or environmental reasons or a combination of all three. Everything outside ourselves is connected to everything inside ourselves. The body follows the mind, and therefore we must treat the whole man in all areas.

> *"The only real mistake is the one from which we learn nothing."*
> —*John Powell*

Little Truths

This section is a mix of writings that didn't make the cut, not because they weren't good enough, but because I just wrote everything down in the order that the information came to me, and the following wasn't a part of it. None of this is in order, and it is meant to be informative in a playful way. I'll start with my prayer, which I say nearly every morning. Sometimes the lessons are so many or so intense for one day that I dare not to ask for more the next day. Please know that I say Buddha even though I am not a Buddhist, and it could be anything one feels comfortable using. Enjoy! I'll end with my very favourite of all:

> *Continue to be intensely curious.*

- My prayer every morning—Dear Buddha, thank you for this day. May the lessons I humbly have to learn come onto my path, that I have wisdom enough to recognize them and be brave enough to undertake them. Shalom.
- "Through meditation we can train our minds so that negative qualities are abandoned and positive qualities are generated and enhanced." —His Holiness the Dalai Lama

- Nothing just happens… Everything happens just.
- Destruction of the world's rainforests has declined by 25 percent during the last decade. —UN Food and Agriculture Organization
- Palm oil plantations are directly responsible for mass clearing of Indonesian rainforests.
- "The future belongs to those who adapt to change." —Charles Darwin
- Avoid eating at least 2 kg of food additives every year by eating organic. —Heaton BFA nutritionist
- When we eat our home-grown food, we become rich not in money but in health, you get successful. Why, because you'll be healthy, happy and healthy. You can't get better than that! —Peter Cundall
- "Nature provides everything we need to protect and maintain our health." —A. Vogel
- 275 Australians develop type-2 diabetes each day, largely due to eating the wrong foods and lack of exercise. —Diabetes Australia, 2012
- There are 28 million child slaves in the world.
- There are no published studies showing GM safety. That is a great concern, since there have been 2 trillion meals consumed made with GM ingredients over the last fifteen years. This does not include GM-fed animal meals.
- 350,000 tonnes of GM soybeans are used in poultry feed, yet the meat does not have to be labelled.
- The way GM chemicals work is that it tears a hole in the insect's intestines and therefore kills it before it reaches adulthood and multiplies. Unfortunately, it did the same to laboratory rats who were fed GM food.

- The three main GM crops used in animal feed are soy, corn and canola. This food is also given to fish.
- Choosing between two evils is still choosing evil. —Jerry Garcia
- Without labelling, it will be very difficult for scientists to trace the source of new illnesses caused by genetically engineered food. —Dr. John Fagan
- The name "arthritis" means inflammation of the joints. Inflammation is caused by lack of sodium in the stomach walls, which therefore causes acidity in the stomach. Eat lots of alkaline foods and exercise. Also avoid nightshade vegetables and drink plenty of water.
- More than 454 million chickens are killed in Australia every year for meat.
- Persistence is stubbornness with a purpose.
- Wisdom is life lessons which have become part of one's being.
- Truth resides in the heart of every man, and it is there that he must seek it in order to be guided by it. —Mahatma Gandhi
- Knowledge comes from learning; wisdom is letting go of what you know.
- Inherent in every problem is its solution.
- One-fourth of what we eat keeps us alive. Three-fourths of what we eat keeps your doctor alive. —Quote from *Food Matters*
- A treat a week is a treat. A treat a day is a habit.
- Pigs are believed to have the intelligence of a three-year-old child.

- Cage-free chickens in Australia raised for meat live in sheds with sixty-thousand other chickens, giving each bird less personal space than one A4- sized piece of paper.
- Every year, seven hundred thousand calves are discarded in Australia alone, labelled a "waste product."—Animals Australia
- Sheep raised for their "ultra-fine" wool live for at least five years locked in a single pen in dark sheds. There is no mental stimulation, and the sheep are on a restricted diet, because starving sheep produce a finer and more valuable wool.
- "Man did not weave the web of life—he is merely a strand in it. Whatever he does to the web he does to himself." —North American leader Chief Seattle, 1854
- It takes more than fifty thousand litres of water to produce one kilogram of beef.
- Over 50 percent of global human-caused greenhouse gases can be attributed to livestock and their by-products.
- Half of the world's fish catch is used to feed herbivores like cattle and pigs.
- People should learn self-responsibility in improving and maintaining their own health.
- Additive 920 is made from animal hair and chicken feathers. —Food and Drug Administration
- Do not cook with olive oil on high heat, as it creates free radicals, as does butter. Coconut oil is the best. Read up on the benefits.
- I recommend slow juicers, which don't heat up and destroy vitamins and minerals. Also, drink your juice straight away.

- I am blood type O. If I would follow a blood type-O diet, I would be riddled with arthritis and asthma at the very least.

- Carnivores sleep most of the day. If you feel sleepy after a meal, most likely you had meat in it.

- Iridology is a science which reveals tissue inflammation and its location in the body. We can look into the eye and see incorrect living, poor diet, mental health, acidity, nervousness and inherited weaknesses and injuries.

- My findings as an iridologist are that people have health struggles because of the strength or weakness of their constitution. Check out your own constitution by looking in the mirror up close. Does your iris have straight lines that go from the pupil to the outside of the iris? Do you have wavy lines with holes or spots? If your iris has straight lines, you have a strong constitution. This means that what you eat or how you live has very little effect on you. Your body can handle a lot. If the lines in your iris are wavy and it looks like some lines split up, making holes, then you have a weak constitution, and you are a person who is deeply affected by your surroundings and by what you eat. People with weak constitutions often have allergies and asthma.

I was blessed with a very weak constitution, which made me responsible for my actions. I always struggled with low energy and asthma, and this led to the study of nutrition. I cannot eat junk, or my joints will ache, I'll be snotty and lethargic. That month, my menstruation will be heavier, more painful and my PMT worse.

211

People with a strong constitution do not get these conditions when they eat junk or acidic foods. They happily eat "whatever" and never get sick. They do get cancer and die eventually, but it is *eventually.*

- Those with a weak constitution are probably healthier than they feel, and those with a strong constitution are probably unhealthier than they feel.
- My parents ate above-average healthy meals. They rarely ate junk food or fast food. They took no medication, didn't smoke, and only my dad had some alcohol now and then. They were not overweight, and they were happy, with little stress. There were no money worries, and both died when they were young. I can't even remember them ever being sick for even one day.

A year after my parents died, my husband and I went to an Andre Rieu concert. As wonderful as it was, it was painfully obvious that the average age there was at least seventy years old. Lots of people were overweight, looked unhealthy, couldn't walk well, and had crutches or wheelchairs. How is it that these people lived longer than my parents? Do other forces influence the length of our time on Earth? My mother had a very small lifeline in her hand, so we always kind of thought she would go early. But really, could it be that once we've learned what we are meant to learn, our time is up?

My mother was also very healthy on an inner level. She always woke up with a song in her heart and found immense happiness inside herself. She was a gardener and loved music; she meditated, read lots of books, and loved her work, her family, friends and her alone time. She always worked on herself. When issues came up, she needed to resolve them because she *needed* to live a life of harmony. She never spoke ill of anyone, and she had a soft approach to life. She was kind but fought for justice. She forgave and loved openly. She gave of her riches, but most importantly, she gave of herself. She wasn't religious but had God within. She never went to church to find God. She believed if God wasn't inside you in the first place, how can you hope to find him in a church or anywhere else? My mother had spiritual peace, and so when her time came, it was for no other reason than that. Her time on this Earth had come to an end, not because she was unhealthy and her poor body gave up, but because she no longer could grow on a spiritual level on this earthly plane. She had learned from life what she had to learn. Her time was up, and she was not scared of death. It was two weeks between her doctor telling her she was not going to survive her cancer and her death. Even while she had cancer, she had more energy than people half her age. She had more get up and go than I. There was no reason to linger. In her living years, she had already told everyone that she loved them and thanked them for enriching her life. She didn't need to ask for forgiveness, and she didn't have to give forgiveness, as all of this had been taken care of while she was living.

- In winter, do yourself a favour and sunbathe. Be in the sun without clothes if you can. This will not only increase your vitamin D naturally, but you also increase your sun protection naturally. Just fifteen minutes is enough. Autumn and spring are also good, but use your own judgement. Never stay in the sun if it is uncomfortable, and never get burned. Our skin will make pigmentation which protects us more when we are in the sun in summertime.

- When we get a cold, it is a way for our bodies to detoxify. This is an elimination process and was caused by the junk food you ate. It is that simple: No junk food/drink, no cold.

- Why do we go to the doctor for a common cold? He is not going to tell you to cut out junk. He'll give you a pill. A patient cured is a customer lost.

- All soybean products such as tofu and soymilk are complete proteins. They contain the essential amino acids plus several other nutrients.

- Vitamin K is necessary for normal blood clotting and maintaining the integrity of the bones. When a baby is born, one of its first needles injected will be filled with synthetic vitamin K. This is not necessary at all because vitamin K appears naturally in all green vegetables. The expectant mothers should be told about this in prenatal classes. They talk about everything else; why not how to prevent a needle being stuck inside your newborn baby? If expectant mothers have lots of greens leading up to the due date, then there is plenty of vitamin K in the breast milk.

- When we are medicine-minded, we have a totally different outlook than if we're nature-minded.

- Your intellect should be a servant, not a master.

- Understand that canned food is no longer a food. Canned food has been boiled, preserved and processed. There is no nutrition left in canned food, making it acidic. Heating food destroys enzymes, vitamins and minerals.

- People who are constipated in the morning have underactive bowels, and they have toxic bacteria which destroys our friendly acidophilus bacteria. This person needs to drink warm water first thing in the morning. During the day, a constipated person needs lots of greens, magnesium and vitamin C. Yellow foods are also laxative. Also, eat lots of raw food, and your bowel will be toned as the sodium goes back to the stomach walls. All this should produce plenty of acidophilus bacteria needed for us to stay regular. Constipated people should never drink coffee, as coffee really irritates the anus area and is known to cause rectal cancer.
- Microwaved food is foodless food. Microwave ovens are excellent to warm up your wheat sack in.
- All salted foods, whether it is salted fish, meat, crackers, nuts and seeds, are constipating foods, as are starchy foods, as is coffee, cheese and chocolate. Burned foods, even smoked foods, vinegars (not organic apple-cider vinegar), pickles, wheat and sugar are some of the worst foods we can have.
- "Pain makes men think. Thinking makes men wise. Wisdom makes life endurable." —John Patrick
- A person who gets all tied up within himself is responsible for tying himself up.
- Tonsillitis is an indication that we have stomach problems, as mucus-producing foods make our digestion sluggish.
- "The richest person knows what it is to walk forward in absolute peace." —Dr. Bernard Jensen

- We need to be aware of the spiritual presence when we make decisions, because life deals out consequences.
- You can produce prostate cancer troubles through fear and anger.
- "When we kill animals, we take in their fear, violence and misery into us, and in us, it also causes fear, misery and violence, which results in illness." —Swami Prakashananda
- Tahini is made of sesame seeds. It is rich in vitamin E, contains protein, zinc and iron. Always buy the unhulled tahini.
- What would you do if you met a healthier version of yourself? How would you feel? What does it take to become that version?
- On the days that you are home, even for the morning or afternoon, do this: drink a couple of glasses of water. Then, when you've gone to the toilet, go and drink two glasses of water straight after. This will become a habit that every time you go to the toilet, you go straight to the kitchen and drink two glasses of water. Please don't flush the toilet every time. Your urine should be light in colour. You should not get hungry as fast and as much when you drink all this water. You should be less bloated, and the next morning, you really can see the difference in your skin. We also lose weight when we do this often enough. Especially for women, this practice is great because you will find that that month, your PMS will be less, you won't have the cravings and there will be less bloating. I do recommend filtering your water and purchasing a prill-bead bag. You need to Google

prill beads for that. Prill beads will alkalise your water, and it lasts forever. Alkalised water is far better than rain or tap-water.

- Every day, we should eat 80 percent alkaline food and 20 percent acidic food. The acidic foods should be alkalising for the stomach, like lemons, which are acidic but alkaline for the stomach, compared to a biscuit, which is an acidic food and also acidic to your stomach.
- You don't have to be your thoughts. If you stop eating sugar, you will stop craving sugar. It takes only three weeks for our taste buds to change.
- "No one is free as long as they are a slave to their body." —Latin phrase
- A "healing crisis" occurs when your body has thrown out lots of toxins and your immunity is up. Your body then goes into a reverse healing pattern of the sicknesses that you've had. The condition does not last long, and you often do not feel sick when you go through a healing crisis.
- "Death in the Western world is largely a food-borne illness." —Dr.Michael Gregar
- Animal protein causes a constant state of inflammation.
- Seventy-eight percent of Australians experience allergies between the ages of fifteen to sixty-four years.
- "When we are no longer able to change a situation, we are challenged to change ourselves." —Victor Frank
- Being healthy is not just being free of illness but a lifestyle.
- "Human beings are the only creatures on earth that claim a God and the only living thing that behaves like it hasn't got one." —Johnny Depp

- Iron foods should be eaten raw whenever possible, as boiling or even soaking causes 46 percent iron loss. Lightly steam iron foods and use the water. These are the highest-iron foods: dulse, kelp, rice bran, greens like spinach, black cherries, unsulphured dried fruits and chlorophyll. Iron can only be absorbed when there is vitamin C in the same food. That is why meat is no good, because it does not contain vitamin C. Iron tablets are highly constipating for our system and are also very bad for our kidneys. Please eat iron foods to get fibre as well, which pills and meat do not contain.

- Our human body is organic and cannot assimilate iron in drug or inorganic form. Nature must manufacture the iron.

- Arthritis sufferers are sensitive to mandarins, oranges and tangerines, even when eaten in small amounts. Arthritis sufferers need magnesium and sodium. Arthritis is not an excess of calcium but a shortage of sodium.

- When there are heart problems, the doctor is likely to put us on a sodium-free diet, but it is better to add potassium for balance, rather than cut out the sodium; otherwise you'll end up with arthritis as well.

- Sodium, potassium, magnesium and silicon are the four alkaline elements that we need to fall back on when we don't feel strong and well enough. All four elements are readily available in foods.

- Avoid eating different kinds of proteins, because plant proteins only require pH 4 acidity, which is durable for our bodies. Dairy needs a pH 2.5 acidity, and that is about our limit. The human stomach can only produce hydrochloric acid of pH 2. Meat needs a pH 1 to be digested, and therefore if you are a frequent meat- and dairy-eater, then your stomach is often in a state of abnormally high pH acidity, which can lead to gastric ulcers.

- Do not eat fruit with other heavier foods. Fruit digests really easily. It will only remain in the stomach for twenty to thirty minutes. If you were to eat bread, dairy or nuts with it, then the fruit will stay in the stomach for as long as it takes to digest these other foods. The fruit will start to ferment and putrefy. This makes a meal acidic, even if it contained alkaline-forming foods. Fruit is best eaten on a empty stomach in the morning. All melons should be eaten by themselves, because their water content is much higher than other fruits; therefore, melons digest quicker. Digestive juices are diluted, so if melon is eaten with other fruit, it also ferments and causes burping and bloating.
- Do not drink with meals, as the liquid dilutes the digestive juices and weakens acidity concentration. Drink water at least twenty minutes before or after a meal. An example of a poor combination is milk on a breakfast cereal.
- Try to commit to eating the right food combinations. You'll find that you will not be bloated, and it means the end to indigestion, wind and burping. 1. Avoid eating acidic foods with starchy foods. Example of these are: orange juice with toast and muesli, or yogurt with fruit and cereal. Starchy foods digest well with salads and lightly steamed vegetables. 2. Avoid proteins and starch in the same meal. This poor combination happens in just

about every meal like meat and potatoes, fish and chips, chicken and corn, rice and chicken, hamburger, cheese sandwich and non-vegan pasta dishes. Eat proteins with lots of greens, and eat starch-rich foods with lots of greens as well. 3. Avoid sugary foods with starch-rich foods because it produces a lot of gas. Sugar on its own will leave the body quickly, but combined with starch, it will sit there fermenting, leading to bloating and gas. Poor combinations include: bread with jam or honey or sweet rice pudding. 4. Avoid sugary foods with protein foods for the same reason. Fruit and nuts is a good example of bad food combinations or cottage cheese with dried fruits. These combinations will cause a lot of wind.

- Breakfast bars are no good because of the wrong food combination, and they have a very long shelf life due to the maltrodextrin.
- There is a connection between lack of sleep and cravings for sugar.
- Fat around your belly pushes on your kidneys, creating diabetes and high blood pressure.
- If you have a glass of alcohol, make the next one water.
- Do not use table salt. Salt is not a food and cannot be digested; instead it preserves. It has no nutritional value and cannot be utilized. Salt is a poison to the heart; it irritates the nervous system, robs the body of calcium and attacks the mucous lining in organs like the lungs.
- Lack of potassium encourages gas generation.
- I've seen acidic irises even though the people ate largely alkaline diets. These people are angry, stressed and

have resentment. Are you one of those people? Learn (even force yourself) to jump out of bed and greet the day with gratitude. Step outside and take a deep breath, looking at all the beauty that is around you. Say, "How lucky am I." Even if this is on a balcony in the middle of the city, you must have this feeling of gratitude because you have chosen this journey. We cannot always do what we like, but we must always like what we do.

- Magnesium contributes to the alkalinity of the body, making the body more flexible.
- Twelve hundred pigs are slaughtered per hour in the United States, and in Canada it is eight hundred per hour.
- Supermarket apples are losing their seeds. Seeds are the lungs of a fruit. Seeds are a life force; without seeds, we eat foodless food.
- In the United States in 2009, the population was 3 percent vegan, and in 2011, it was 5 percent vegan.
- "It is not happy people who are thankful. It is thankful people who are happy." —David Murray
- The state of your life is nothing more than the reflection of your state of mind.
- Every day, more than 170 million land animals are killed for food.
- Just because you've been programmed to believe something, that doesn't make it true.
- "We are not held back by the love we didn't receive in the past, but by the love we're not extending in the present." —Marianne Williamson
- We must change. Change is our journey.

- "Those who mind don't matter, and those who matter don't mind." —Bernard M. Baruch
- Thyroid disturbances come from stress in sadness. Balance the nerves and mental state. People with thyroid problems cannot have ice or cold drinks, because this brings more stress to the body.
- If we are constantly in a state of stress, our digestion will suffer. Irritable bowel syndrome will develop as a result.
- The global livestock industry is responsible for more greenhouse-gas emissions than all planes, trains, and cars in the world combined. Livestock industries produce 130 times that of the entire human population.
- The spiritual becomes before the mental and physical.
- Cleverness divides, while natural intelligence always includes.
- Veganism represents and promotes all life to the fullest and to the highest level of consciousness.
- It baffles me that truly kind and caring people can be kind to their own dog or cat but so indifferent to the suffering of other animal beings. According to a new study by European researchers, meat-eaters have less empathy than vegetarians. The researchers recruited sixty-two volunteers: twenty meat-eaters, twenty-one vegans, and twenty-one vegetarians, and placed them into an MRI machine, while showing them a series of random pictures. The MRI scans revealed that when observing animal or human suffering, the "empathy-related" areas of the brain were more active among vegetarians and vegans. The researchers even found that there are certain brainwaves and areas that only vegans

and vegetarians seem to activate when witnessing a suffering animal or human. The vegetarians and vegans also scored significantly higher on an empathy-quotient questionnaire than the meat-eaters did. This study wasn't done to make vegans and vegetarians look more self-righteous, but they were doing a study on making compassionate choices and who is more capable of making them. —Daniel R. Rowes of *Psychology Today*

- Our energy is the same as our earth's energy. After December 23, 2012, our vibrational energy shifted to a higher frequency. (The shift started in 2011, when every soul energy got opportunities to open up to growth, and this intensified as it got closer to 2012.) Even our physical bodies can vibrate at a higher frequency. Also, we will see each other in a different light. We will appreciate and recognise god-light itself as our consciousness will expand. As our perception changes, we will find spiritualism normal, without all the "airy-fairy" stigma that use to be attached to spiritualism. Our Earth is changing because our consciousness has changed to a higher frequency. We cannot judge those who do not know or feel this connection to growth. The "light" is always there, and it is only time which will have people connect to it. In time, there are many lessons which are opportunities for us to learn. These lessons can be perceived as negative events, and this creates fear. This is the wrong way to go about growth. Growth is all about the love that you get when you have learned the lesson. That is our universal law—love! Everything that is not love is a lack of love. Fear is a lack of love.

Fear creates control. Fear creates war and disharmony and greed. Once a fear-based problem is embraced by love, then the problem is solved. It is really as simple as that, since there is enough food for everyone on the planet, since there is more than enough money on the planet, there is more than enough beauty on the planet for us to live without war, famine and destruction. This is where the saying comes from: "For as long as men massacre animals, they will kill each other. Indeed, he who sows the seed of murder and pain cannot reap joy and love" —Pythagoras (sixth century BC). Once we stop eating the blood of another, we can understand how to be peaceful. Once we know how to be peaceful, we can create peaceful governments. As you can see from the saying, we are very slow to acknowledge this perception.

- We are God-light; we just don't know it yet. We must be in awe of ourselves, the way our higher selves see us.
- Allergies are created from an emotional state, so the body will be affected.
- Fast food and junk food are addictive. Acknowledge that you are having a hard time being addicted to fast food. Look up "tapping" on Google; this method will help.
- Eating meat is an ethical and moral issue, and not to eat it is an insult to our mothers.

They say it takes three weeks to break a habit. Let's presume this is true. Why is it, then, that we are not all non-smokers, fit and healthy, if breaking a habit was so easy. Why does it not last? Let's take John. John is your typical Aussie man who drinks a little too much and wants to limit it a bit and become fitter. The first week goes great. John gets up most mornings to go for a brisk walk and he has only one beer with his mates. He feels great. The second week also goes well, but that weekend, John has his usual amount of beers. It is a friend's fortieth, and that only happens once, so you have to live it up for this special occasion. Besides that, John feels he has been "good" all week, and so he deserves a bit of fun. The third week, John doesn't feel so well after his big weekend, and as a result, he doesn't get out of bed early and doesn't go for his walk. There is always tomorrow.

We all recognize this scenario. So why does this happen? Did you know that life will put these special occasions on our path on purpose? It is an opportunity to grow. Do we go to our familiar drinking hole and have just one beer, or do we do what we always do when we are with these people in this situation? See how this scenario relates to weight loss or any concerning behaviour as well? Are we even aware of our destructive habits?

John fell back into the old pattern of drinking with his mates and not exercising. Why is that? It is because John never changed the person he was. He still was an excessive beer drinker who just drank less and walked in the mornings. He never changed how he viewed himself. To change, we must change our vicious circle. To break any habit—let's say smoking—we first must become healthier. We must clean out our systems first, because our bodies will crave the old habit for as long as its toxins are inside of us. With cravings, our ego will overrule our reason for giving up our destructive behaviour and therefore our new lifestyle and go back to where we are comfortable.

When we clean out our systems, perhaps by going on a juice fast for a few days, we increase our level of vibration. Our brains will also be cleansed, and we view everything more clearly than before. Once we have cleaned out our systems, then the whole "change to a better lifestyle" is easier. We will not crave the smokes as much, and there is less talk from our ego.

So, cleaning out our systems really just means eating lots of fruits and greens, lots of raw stuff, drinking more water, and cutting down on processed foods, fats and sugars. Why do we cut out these foods? Because they are dead foods. There is no life energy in these foods whatsoever. They are always acidic, which goes against what we need in order to raise our level of vibration and become healthier. Alkaline foods and alkaline-forming foods are alive foods. Alkaline foods also help to rid the body of toxins. Getting rid of toxins is the link that will stop an abusive vicious circle. In order to break a habit, we must clean out our systems first.

Let's go back to John, and let's go back two weeks earlier, before John's walking routine started. This time, John views himself first as a healthy, fit person, and so he cleans out his system. He eats carrots (with the skin on) and apples (also with the skin on), drinks lots of water, and mentally prepares himself for the change he is about to make. He imagines himself walking and being healthier. In this state, it is much easier to break a habit. His cravings for beer will be lessened, and his energy level will be increased. He might even have lost weight in the meantime, because junk food during the week and the barbeque on the weekend is not part of a healthy and fit person. Mentally, he is better prepared, and when that first Monday morning came around, it really wasn't that much of a change. He probably looked forward to it more, because he had been sleeping a lot better and therefore, he was rested when it came to jumping out of bed and exercising. This is his new "vicious circle." Eat healthy, feel better, have more energy, sleep better, get better rest, get up early to exercise, working up a healthy appetite.

A clean, vibrant body goes with an optimistic, happy mind. John has a far better chance to break a habit in three weeks. He will naturally not feel like much beer, and instead of steak, potatoes with gravy and a piece of white bread, John now eats salad and veggies. By doing this, John now has raised his vibrational level. Of course, he will be tested whether he "owns" the new pattern or not. So, the fortieth comes around, and John goes to the old, familiar drinking hole, which now stinks of old, stale beer. (Cleaning out toxins improves our sense of smell.) He decides to have a beer but drinks water the rest of the night, while his mates get drunker and sillier. Even though he enjoys their company for a bit, he'd rather go home at a reasonable time than doing an all-nighter.

I believe this theory goes for all bad habits that we want to change. There have been several cases where a temperamental person decided to get healthy. When eating healthier, the body and mind are cleared of toxins, and these individuals felt a lot differently. As soon as toxins had left the brain, these individuals felt happier and more reasonable.

- With eating healthier foods comes the study of healthier foods. With learning about eating healthy comes the notion that we are responsible for our own behaviour.

With being responsible for our own actions comes change in behaviour. We learn about change and its rewards waiting for us as soon as we own that change. All this raises the level of vibration. Everything living has a living vibration, an aura. All junk food has no vibration or aura because the food is dead. Eating dead food leads to toxins, which leads to lower personal vibration, which leads to poorer physical and spiritual immunity. We get sick, which leads to medication, which is more toxins, which leads to lower immunity and brain fog. If you are serious about changing an unfavourable habit, then before you give it up, change your diet first for at least two weeks beforehand, and the changeover will go a lot smoother.

- All foods grown from this earth's soil have this living vibration. When we grow our own food, these foods can last for years. Imagine eating food and not actually killing it to eat it. An apple tree must have its apples picked and eaten in order to grow and stay strong. We do not kill fruit trees by eating their fruit, and every food produces more than enough seeds for the propagation of generations to come.

- "Think globally, act locally." —Patrick Geddes

- Figs are extremely high in calcium. Sesame seeds are also very high. Molasses is also very high in calcium and iron as well.

- Coffee reduces the body's ability to absorb iron.

- Spend your money on good, organic food, because if you don't spend it on good food you'll be spending it on doctors. Doctors make a living on the mistakes we make in our kitchen and what we eat.

- Cholesterol comes from eggs, meat and milk products.
- The best defence against cancer is your own body's resistance to it.
- The teeth of carnivorous animals have 5 percent magnesium phosphate, which enables them to crush and grind bones of their pray. Humans have 1 percent magnesium phosphate.
- Yellow foods indicate magnesium, like corn, yellow squash and bananas. All laxative foods in nature are yellow.
- High-sodium foods like celery and parsley alkalise the stomach.
- Potassium is needed in the muscle structure.
- Mean people lack iodine.
- Within us is a quiet place where we can meet with God to seek the wisdom we need for right living and understanding. In there lies the foundation of truth. This truth comes from the soul.
- White sugar leaches calcium from the body, causes a vitamin B-complex deficiency and causes reduced hunger for proper food. Deficiencies lead to nervous problems, nervous breakdowns and mental illness, heart problems, constipation, mouth and skin disorders. Artificial sweeteners contribute nothing nutritionally at all to the body and have been proven harmful.
- Calcium should always be with phosphorus, as calcium cannot be used in the body without phosphorus. Tahini is a great food that contains both.

- We only have so much digestive juice to take care of a meal. If you eat too much, it is very hard on your digestive system, because the surplus depletes your energy.
- Melons should be eaten by themselves and twenty minutes before or after other food. Please eat their seeds, as they have chlorophyll, vitamin K and iron in them, which makes them good for kidney trouble, hypertension and high blood pressure.
- Meat and potatoes are a very poor combination. Meat should be eaten with lots of greens, and potatoes should be eaten with lots of greens.
- The pulp in an orange is the calcium that neutralizes the acids. Orange juice does not have pulp and ends up a very acidic drink. Vitamin C diminishes with oxygen, light and time, so the orange juice you buy has no nutritional value and is very acidic for your body.
- Acid irritates the lining of the stomach and bowel.
- Salt is not a food and contributes to the hardening of the arteries.
- Black pepper is a liver irritant.
- Best starches: millet, brown rice, rye, yellow cornmeal. Second best: buckwheat, oats, barley, soybeans and baked potato. Have these once in a while.
- Best proteins: Seeds and nuts, unhulled tahini, alfalfa and beans. Almonds are the only nuts that are alkaline. Brazil nuts and walnuts are high in manganese, which is a memory element.
- An arthritic person should drink distilled water or alkaline water. Never drink coffee or tea or alcohol. Drink potato broth.

- Doctors are yet to find a disease caused by veganism.
- Sodium foods are cooling and great to eat in summertime to cool yourself down. Cucumber, pineapple, lettuce, parsley, okra, strawberries and celery are sodium foods.
- Sulphur foods create heat in the body. Broccoli, cauliflower, cabbage and kale are sulphur foods.
- Malva is considered a weed and is very high in vitamin A.
- Do not use white flour. Find another alternative.
- Ginseng, gotu kola, fo-ti-tieng and sage promote longevity.
- Circles under the eyes mean lack of iron in the blood.
- For a sore throat, drink chlorophyll. If you have a cough as well, cut up an organic onion in small, diced pieces and put this in a mug. Cover with organic honey. Let it sit for at least one hour and up to two hours. With a spoon, push down on the onion and let the liquid fill the spoon. Slowly drink this. It is very soothing for the throat, and it helps the cough.
- For earache, put strong garlic-juice drops into the ear a few times a day. Hardening of the ear comes from too much salt. Sodium foods and slant-board exercises and lots of vitamin C help.
- Hair—Lecithin is good for hair, as is oat-straw tea and shave-grass tea and avocado. These foods are also brain foods because of the silicon in them.
- Valerian and chamomile tea are good if you can't sleep.
- People who snore should not have heavy starches.
- Foods high in iron are good for the liver. Dandelion and chlorophyll is good.
- Sprouts like alfalfa are great for the nerves. Include them in your foods often.

- For poor memory, eat sodium foods and manganese, vitamin B complex and do slant-board exercises.
- Heart—Good for the heart are chlorophyll, vitamin E and hawthorn tea. Avoid beef.
- Anaemic condition—The best iron foods are black cherries and blackberries, all greens, watercress and any other foods that contain silicon, iron and sodium.
- Haemorrhoids—Increase iron intake, vitamin K and nettle tea.
- Kidney trouble—cut out citrus, increase water, drink organic homemade vegetable juice, and drink organic watermelon juice with seed and skin if the fruit is young.
- Lungs—For healthy lungs, we must eat non-catarrhal foods, to get rid of excess catarrh in the lungs. Avoid milk, wheat and citrus. Eat vegetables and drink chlorophyll.
- Piles happen when we eat the wrong combination of foods over a period of time.
- Man gladly believes what he wishes to be true and defends these beliefs so strongly that eventually his laws will be written this way. In the end, they believe their own wrongs and teach their children these laws.
- Did you know that it takes thirty-two glasses of water to neutralize the acid in one can of cola?
- 1.7 million Australians are living with diabetes, and 275 people develop the disease every day. —Diabetes Australia
- The peanut is not a nut but a legume. Peanuts are one of the world's oldest crops.

- Spinach is rich in lutein and zeaxanthin, which helps to slow down macular degeneration of the eye and maintain your eyesight.
- Zinc competes with iron, and it is one or the other that your body can absorb.
- When we die, our bodies turn acidic very quickly so that they can break down. When we eat acidic foods, the body becomes acidic, and the body breaks down while we are alive.
- Alkaline fruits include watermelon, apricots, figs, cantaloupe, apples, bananas, pineapples, nectarines and blackberries.
- Alkaline veggies include sea vegetables like nori, kelp, dulse and wakame, broccoli, carrots, cabbage, cauliflower, celery, parsley, eggplant, squash, turnips and dark leafy greens like kale and spinach.
- Acidic foods and drinks include all animal proteins, beer, coffee, tea, and all carbonated drinks.
- Iodine is a very important mineral for the thyroid and helps the thyroid to function fully. However, the thyroid cannot absorb or get access to the iodine if the body's pH is not alkaline. Thyroid problems have been linked to arthritis, cancer, depression, heart attacks, obesity and fatigue.
- If you have lemon juice, have it first thing in the morning with warm water. The magnesium in lemons is highly anti-acid and converts to alkalinise the stomach. This process only happens first thing in the morning. Lemon juice at any other time of the day will be converted to an acidic state. An alternative to warm lemon juice first thing in the morning is organic apple-cider vinegar.

- "Now I can look at you in peace; I don't eat you anymore." —Franz Kafka
- "If slaughterhouses had glass walls, everyone would be a vegetarian." —Paul and Linda McCartney
- "Peace cannot be kept by force. It can only be achieved by understanding." —Albert Einstein.
- "Man is the only animal that can remain on friendly terms with the victims he intends to eat until he eats them." — Samuel Butler, *Note-Books,* 1912
- "I just could not stand the idea of eating meat. People's general awareness is getting much better, even down to buying a pint of milk: the fact that the calves are actually killed so that the milk doesn't go to them but to us cannot really be right, and if you have seen a cow in a state of extreme distress because it cannot understand why its calf isn't by, it can make you think a lot." —Kate Bush
- "People think of animals as if they were vegetables, and that is not right. We have to change the way people think about animals. I encourage the Tibetan people and all people to move toward a vegetarian diet that doesn't cause suffering." —The Dalai Lama
- Putrefaction in meat-eaters is evidenced by bad breath, heartburn, and the foul stool and odorous emissions— absent in vegetarians. *—Raw Food Explained*
- "How can you eat anything with a heart as big as yours?" —Kelsey Kimler
- "We could never learn to be brave and patient if there were only joy in the world." —Helen Keller
- "Meat is the dead body of someone who wanted to live." *—Animalequality.org*

- "It's pretty amazing to wake up every morning, knowing that every decision I make is to cause as little harm as possible. It's a pretty fantastic way to live." —Colleen Patrick-Goudreau

- "We do not experience things as they really are! We experience things only through a filter and that filter determines what information will enter our awareness and what will be rejected. If we change the filter (our belief system), then we automatically experience the world in a completely different way." —David Wolfe

- "If you knew how meat was made, you'd probably lose your lunch." —k.d. lang

- "Health is not valued until sickness comes." —Thomas Fuller

- "May our daily choices be a reflection of our deepest values, and may we use our voices to speak for those who need us most, those who have no voice, those who have no choice." —Colleen Patrick-Goudreau

- "A vegan driving a hummer contributes less greenhouse-gas emissions than a meat-eater riding a bicycle." —Captain Paul Watson

- Aura is the light surrounding our alive body. Some say it is the soul itself, because when we die, that light goes out.

- Cow's milk is very poor in iron, but a dairy farmer will tell you that it is good for you, even though one teaspoon of cow's milk contains more than 40 million germs. These are not the kind of germs we need. A cheese-maker will always say that cheese is good for you. A butcher with a red-capillary face and red nose will say meat is good for you, and a goat-soap maker will tell you that goat soap is the best around. Please use your own judgement, and look at who is releasing statistics. It is never an independent company.

- If doctors did more nutritional educating, they would do less medicating.
- Without sufficient iodine and vitamin D, calcium cannot be properly used in the body. Without vitamin B12 and vitamin C, iron cannot be assimilated. That is why we need such a large variety of organic foods.
- Vitamins are not as necessary in the body as minerals. Minerals control and hold the vitamins in the body. It is like minerals build the body and vitamins run the body.
- The four most important chemical elements are calcium, iodine, sodium and silicon.
- The liver is the organ which breaks down toxins. When the liver is not functioning properly, toxins may be converted to the brain, causing "brain fog."
- Caffeinated foods and drinks and hot spices make us agitated, nervous and restless. Prune and celery juice are a wonderful nerve food.
- Omega 3 from fish is there because of the algae they eat.
- The two paths of opportunity—which one will you take? Do we go back to what we know is familiar, or do we venture into the unknown? It takes courage to change, but how do we know that we need to change? We need to change when what we are doing is not working for us anymore.
- We must learn to listen to that little voice inside of us. We can only listen when we are still. We shouldn't talk

so much unless we are being paid for it. People who talk too much don't listen to themselves. Be still, create stillness, try meditation, and in your stillness, you will find the right path to take. We cannot live well without happiness, and even though happiness is hard to find within us, it is impossible to find it anywhere else.

Why are we happy to run ourselves down to the state of sickness? Is it because we want to work long hours to buy the bigger house, second car or overseas holiday? We must enjoy our work. It is okay to work extremely hard for what you want to achieve, but you must be happy within yourself to do this without getting sick. So, what is really important then? In your stillness, you will find your answer. If you want financial riches but don't have inner happiness, then you are inviting ulcers into your life as well.

Of course, we can be rich and happy, but it wouldn't matter whether you are financially well off, as long as you have inner happiness. If you really cannot live without luxuries, no matter what, then it is your ego you are listening to. Our ego is a show pony that is busy, noisy, creates routine and makes us think that everything that is available outside ourselves is important. That is why it is so important to be quiet, peaceful and humble. Even when we don't listen to our inner self for a while, that voice will just lay dormant, but it never goes away. That inner voice just waits for life's lessons to knock on your door, because it knows it is just a matter of time.

Over time, we should get better and better at identifying the lesson and take the right path. In fact, we should recognize when we are in a "quiet karma time" as well. Enjoy this time, as it will not last. This is a lesson in itself. We catch ourselves saying that life is running very smoothly right now. Not wanting for more, being satisfied and being aware of it is happiness. And then something shifts, sometimes small and sometimes huge, like a death of a loved one. If we can recognize the need for the shift, then we will not fight against it. We will grieve, but we'll go with the flow.

Sometimes, especially with death, it is very hard to look for an upside, and I will never accept that there is an upside to the loss of a child. I think that happiness from that moment onwards is felt with a broken heart. Shifts in life will make us think, and maybe we'll become more spiritual; then there is a shift in the person's thinking. When we are confronted with a situation that makes us think, we will want to be quiet. All this will lead to awareness, and awareness leads to connection and compassion. This is when people say "enjoy the journey and don't look back," because if you look back at situations, you will miss the doors opening in front of you.

- Chocolate cravings are a sign of magnesium deficiency and will fade when sufficient magnesium is given.
- One needs magnesium utilization of calcium for bone-building. Calcium should be deposited in soft tissue, rather than in the bones. This experiment was described in *Metabolic Aspects of Health:* A calcium-rich diet was given to chickens, with the result that they laid thin, weak-shelled eggs. Then the chickens were given no calcium but a diet of magnesium, silica and other minerals. The eggs that came from this had calcium-rich shells, which proves that the Animal Kingdom is

capable of transforming magnesium and other minerals into calcium. This also explains why a vegetable-rich diet builds strong teeth and bones. So it is magnesium that is essential for the development of healthy bones.

- Grains are the enemy of bones.
- Table salt causes large amounts of calcium loss through the excretion of urine.
- In 2011, many were shocked to see footage from a Hawkesbury Valley abattoir showing scenes of extreme cruelty. The footage showed a worker bashing a pig over the head with a metal bar and sheep being hung by their legs while still fully conscious. The abattoir was fined $5,200. This is outrageous, and unfortunately there were many similar incidents. In all ten abattoirs which were visited, animal-welfare breaches were uncovered. Pigs, cows, chickens and sheep were not stunned properly, and dismembering happened while animals were conscious. As shocking as it is, this is the reality as long as we make the decision to eat animal beings.
- When a person experiences dizziness, he or she needs sodium chloride.
- A person with a dry mouth needs sodium chloride.
- A person with dry skin needs sodium and chloride.
- A person who has menstrual disorders lacks iron.
- A person with nosebleeds or other haemorrhages lacks calcium.
- When ears are itching and flaky, phosphorus is lacking.
- Paths of opportunity—Have you ever known a person to leave an abusive relationship, only to go to another abusive relationship? Why does this happen? It happens

because the level of vibration did not change in the meantime, and so the person is attracted to the familiarity of that level. Every time we leave an unhealthy situation, we have the opportunity to see this as a chance to change and get on to the path of opportunity. Often this comes with feelings of uncertainty, and that's why we often go back to what we know, rather than venturing into the unknown. It takes courage to change, no matter how small the change. We need courage to let go of what is familiar. We know it is time to change because what we are used to isn't working for us anymore. Suddenly the pasta and steaks you've had your whole life don't sit right in your gut anymore. "Changes in life" will find us, and they will knock on our door. It is not the other way around. Life will always present changes to us, and it is up to us to take the path of opportunity.

- For those who are blessed enough to know meditation, you know that this is the time to listen for the answers which are inside of you already. Being still or going for a walk is also good to clear our minds, because it is when we are still that we get the opportunity to listen. This happens when we stop our routine and stop thinking for a moment. As long as the TV is going or the radio is on, we don't hear life's lessons knocking on the door. Life has a tendency to keep us busy in a world of escapism. Why is it that we get sick when we go on holidays? Is it because when life's lessons knocked on the door to tell us to take it easy, that we are living on our reserves, and to take up golf or yoga, we ignored it? We must listen, and we can only listen when we are still. We need to create that stillness. Don't talk so much. Don't do so much. Don't work so much. Create an environment that encourages well-being of the soul and the physical body. What is really important? In your stillness, you will find the answer. It is then up to you to either listen or to ignore it. Are you going to ignore the path of opportunity?

The vine of inner happiness can lay dormant for a long time, waiting for the lessons in life to knock on your door and for you to choose the path that is going to fill you up internally rather than externally. When a problem arises, the sand starts pouring from the top to the bottom. Do not allow this to happen; turn the hourglass around. It is important that you learn to see things as positive as quickly as possible. Why? Because if we keep looking back at a situation, we'll miss the doors opening in front of us. This is a big shift in a person's thinking. It forces us to stop being victims, and not everyone likes that. Next time something happens that pisses you off, be aware of "victimism" and turn that around to wishing the situation well and letting go.

- At the end of the day, if you must eat animal beings, spare a moment thinking about their journey to your table. Try to feel what the animal being must have felt and what emotions it might have had. Ask forgiveness for removing its life. No, not to the animal, but say sorry to yourself, because on so many levels you are letting your own higher self down. Remember, dying is never as bad as killing.

Spiritually—we can no longer eat the flesh of another.

Environmentally—we can no longer sustain meat eating.

Health—it is proven that vegans do not have the health problems that meat-eaters have.

Ethically—be responsible for your actions, and if it involves the killing of an animal being, think twice and do not use excuses like, "God provided animals for our use." God also gave us good and evil, and with that, *free* will. Furthermore, there is plenty of other food for us to eat.

Be the best you can be.

Sandra's Super Banana Milkshake Recipe

Blender
1 banana per person

Slice bananas into blender and fill it up with any of the following liquids equal to the level of the bananas in blender (making sure it is all organic): rice milk, almond milk, soymilk, or any nut milk. Please feel free to use water as well, but *never ever* use animal milk.

Organic unhulled tahini—pour in the equivalent of a couple of tablespoons. Macro from Woolworth's is a good one. Melrose have a good one as well, but it is more expensive.

LSA mix—this is ground linseed, almond and sunflower seeds. Add one heaping tablespoon into blender.

Organic Golden Flaxmeal from Melrose—this can be purchased at Woolworth's as well.

Super Greens from Synergy—this is spirulina, chlorella, barley grass and wheatgrass. Please note: it is the grass bit and not the wheat bit that they use for this green mixture. Put a heaping tablespoon into the blender

BeetAgreens from Wonderfoods—this can be purchased at the health-food shop. Put a heaping tablespoon into the blender.

Omega balance—this is your omega 3, 6 and 9. Please note that fish and krill oil only have omega 3, and proper absorption can only occur with the correct ratio of 3, 6 and 9. Fish and krill oil are also acidic and therefore do your body more harm than good.

Melrose Vitamin C Sodium Ascorbate Powder—put one heaping teaspoon into the blender.

Blend all together for about ten seconds or until everything is mixed. I tend not to overblend, as it destroys fragile nutrients, and I find the mixture thickens up with too much blending. Pour and drink straight away, as light and oxygen also destroy vital nutrients.

Recommended Books

Veganist by Kathy Freston
The Lean by Kathy Freston
The 30-Day Vegan Challenge by Colleen Patrick-Goudreau
Fit for Life by Harvey Diamond and Marilyn Diamond

Recommended Documentaries

Forks Over Knives by Lee Fulkerson

Food, Inc. by Robert Kenner

Earthlings by Shaun Monson

Devour the Earth (1995)

Meet Your Meat (2002)

Peaceable Kingdom (2004)

A Sacred Duty (2007)

A Delicate Balance – The Truth (2008)

Simply Raw: Reversing Diabetes in 30 Days (2009)

Fat, Sick and Nearly Dead (2010)

Planeat (2010)

Vegucated (2011)

Unsupersize Me (2013)

Meat the Truth (2008)

Recommended Websites

www.veganaustralia.net
www.vegsoc.org.au
www.vegsource.com

Famous Vegans

Ellen DeGeneres
Portia DiRossi
Alec Baldwin
Justin Bieber
Usher
Rosie O'Donnell
Kristen Bell
Pamela Anderson
Russell Brand
Lea Michele
Carrie Underwood
Paul McCartney
Olivia Wilde
Alicia Silverstone
Joaquin Phoenix
Dennis Kucinich
Bill Clinton
Brad Pitt
Ted Danson
Mike Tyson

Anthony Kiedis
Anne Hathaway
Dax Shepard
Bryan Adams
Emily Deschanel
James Cromwell
Betty White
KD Lang
Jenny McCarthy
Petra Nemcova
Ruben Studdard
Sandra Oh
Jessica Chastain
Tobey Maguire
Robin Gibb
Carl Lewis
Chickezie
Chrissie Hynde
Biz Stone
Chelsea Clinton

Russell Simmons

Woody Harrelson

Natalie Portman

Stella McCartney

Daryl Hannah

Jane Lynch

Fran Drescher

Venus and Serena Williams

References

Potassium Ring, page 52: *The Chemistry of Man,* Dr. Bernard Jensen, page 295.

Iridology Chart, page 69: Given to me by Dr. Bernard Jensen, who is the founder and designer of this chart.

Tofu and Tempeh Chart, page 85: Designed by Dierk Kimler. Information from Ijayhealth and forkstofeet.

Bowels, page 91: Designed by Dierk Kimler. Information from *The Atlantean Conspiracy.*

Humans Are Biologically Herbivorous, page 95: *The Comparative Anatomy of Eating* by Milton R. Mills, MD.

Carnivore, Herbivore, Human Chart, page 96: Published by Brian Wong. Designed by Dierk Kimler. Information from *www. detox.net.*

The Raw Food Pyramid, page 146: Used with the permission of Audra Mott, "Rawkin Good Food by Audra," *www. rawkingoodfoodbyaudra.com,* Seal Beach, CA, 2013.

[1] Chemical Elements (pages 37–51) includes information taken from: Bernard Jensen, PhD, *The Chemistry of Man—Volume II, "Man" Series* (Escondido, Bernard Jensen, Publisher, 1983) pages 112–363.

[2] Based on my own research.

[3] "Osteoporosis: Fast Facts." National Osteoporosis Foundation. "Milk, dietary calcium, and bone fractures in women: a 12-year prospective study." Am. J. Public Health, 1997; 87:992–97.

[4] Animals Australia: Dairy Cows Fact Sheet.

[5] FoodBev Media: Shaun Weston Aug 2010 in Cooler Innovation Magazine.

[6] Foodwatch, Organic: "A Climate Saviour? The foodwatch report on the greenhouse effect of conventional and organic farming in Germany, based on the study 'The Impact of German Agriculture on the Climate'" by the Institute for Ecological Economy Research (IÖW), 2009.

[7 and 8] Gail A. Eisnitz, *Slaughterhouse—The Shocking Story of Greed, Neglect, and Inhumane Treatment Inside the U.S. Meat Industry.* (New York, Prometheus Books, 1997).

About the Author

Sandra Kimler (Spykers) was born in Rotterdam, the Netherlands, in 1964. She immigrated to Australia with her family in 1978, settling in the Kiewa Valley in Victoria. Through her mother, Hennie Spykers-Hersman's influence, Sandra received qualifications in nutrition and iridology, studying the teachings of Dr. Bernard Jensen. Having been a vegetarian from a young age, today Sandra is a vegan, passionate animal-rights activist, successful businesswoman and mother of three wonderful children.

Sandra currently resides near Byron Bay in northern NSW, Australia.

If you would like to contact Sandra:
sandrakimler@gmail.com